SONNY BUBBA'S
Southern Fried
Semi-low Calorie

SONNY BUBBA'S
Southern Fried Semi-low Calorie Cookbook

Sonny Bubba Ferguson

RUTLEDGE HILL PRESS
Nashville, Tennessee

Published in Nashville, Tennessee, by Rutledge Hill Press, Inc., 513 Third Avenue South, Nashville, Tennessee 37210.

Typography by Bailey Typography, Inc., Nashville, Tennessee.

Library of Congress Cataloging-in-Publication Data

Ferguson, Sonny Bubba, 1943-
    [Southern fried semi-low calorie cookbook]
    Sonny Bubba's southern fried semi-low calorie cookbook / Sonny Bubba Ferguson.
        p.   cm.
    ISBN 1-55853-034-7
    1. Cookery, American—Southern style.   I. Title.   II. Title: Southern fried semi-low calorie cookbook.
TX715.2.S68F47   1989
641.5975—dc20   89-10839
                                                                                        CIP

Printed in the United States of America
1 2 3 4 5 6 7 8 — 94 93 92 91 90 89

Contents

Introduction

Real Men Don't Go On Diets

I realize that diet is an unpleasant word in many households, particularly south of the Mason-Dixon line. Diets are what a woman resorts to when she's got to get into a dress for a niece's wedding or attend a high school reunion. Diets are what a man goes on when his doctors tell him he's on the verge of a heart attack or stroke, or his mechanic informs him that the springs on his pickup truck are ruined from hauling heavy loads.

To most red-blooded southern men and women, diets mean water-packed tuna fish and bean sprouts, lots of lettuce and carrots, and no barbecue.

New Yorkers may actually like tuna vinaigrette, and folks in San Francisco may have a taste for tofu, but down South we have to have our Brunswick stew, corn bread, and fried green tomatoes.

I know. I've tried everything from the Scarsdale Diet to the Root Beer and Burrito Diet. They all work—as long as you stay on them. It's staying on them that's the problem.

If you've been raised, like I have, by a mama and two aunts who think a light snack is fried chicken, potato salad, rice and gravy, green beans, and corn on the cob, then you've got a severe handicap to overcome. You can only go so long without a pork chop, a bowl of Brunswick stew, or a mess of fried okra.

Not long ago I was congratulating myself on having

lasted for three weeks without dieting. I'd made two visits to Mama's and three trips to the Brookton All-You-Can-Eat Catfish School. That weekend I dug into the back of my closet and found my favorite orange and green plaid double knit pants that my wife keeps hiding from me.

They were too small, but I knew the problem immediately. My wife had stored them in the attic over the winter, and they had shrunk. So had my yellow Bermuda shorts and my bikini bathing suit that I used to wear to sunbathe in the backyard until the woman next door called the police.

I pointed this out to my wife that night at supper, as I carefully spooned some tomato gravy over a chunk of meat loaf.

"You've gained weight," she said, chewing daintily on a stalk of steamed broccoli.

"Maybe a pound or two," I said, reaching for the mashed potatoes.

"A pound or two?" she laughed. "If you gain any more weight, the TV people will ask you to do stunts on 'Jake and the Fat Man.'"

I disagreed, of course. I'm not that fat. On the weight scale, I fall somewhere between Raymond Burr and Burl Ives, although that sounds kind of painful.

"Let's face it," she said, pulling the basket of rolls out of reach. "You need to go on another diet."

I was about to protest when she started telling me about a talk show hostess who had lost more than sixty pounds on the Okra Diet. At least that's what I thought she said. Two weeks and ten pounds of boiled okra later, I knew something was wrong. I kept sliding out of my chair.

"It's the Oprah Diet, not the Okra Diet," my wife said when I complained about my problem. "Oprah Winfrey lost weight on a liquid diet."

"Kind of like Roy Bill's?" I asked. Roy Bill has consumed more light beer than the guys on the Miller commercials.

"No, dummy," she laughed affectionately. "It's liquid protein, and you have to be under a doctor's supervision."

That didn't sound nearly as appealing as Roy Bill's

menu, so I decided then and there that I would make up my own diet. My diet would have good things to eat, like barbecue and Brunswick stew and fried chicken and corn bread. That was the kind of food a good ole boy or good ole girl could eat indefinitely. With a few changes, there was no reason southern food couldn't be as healthy as any other kind—and twice as tasty.

The wives I talked to agreed. No matter how good a diet was, if their husbands didn't stick to it and sneaked off to Po Folks or for a six-pack and a half-pound of fried pork rinds, it didn't do any good.

"I love Roy Bill dearly," his wife, Eleanor, said when I told her about my project, "but he acts so pitiful if I don't cook him up a batch of biscuits on Sunday morning. It was all I could do to wean him off fried fatback. He said real men don't go on diets."

I used to believe the same thing. Then I noticed how many real men were being carried out of their houses feet first in the prime of life. I didn't expect to change decades of bad eating habits overnight, but I knew there ought to be a way to make some inroads.

Even Roy Bill was interested. "If you can come up with a diet that has barbecue, Brunswick stew, and fried okra, I'll do it," he said, eating his third Penrose pickled hot sausage with his beer.

"No alcohol except on cheatin' days," I said.

"That's all right."

"And fried foods no more than once a week."

"I can do that."

I smiled. The first hurdle to *Sonny Bubba's Southern Fried Semi-low Calorie Cookbook and Weight-loss Guide* had been cleared.

PART ONE:

The Sonny Bubba Weight-loss Guide

ONE

Blame It on Scarlett

The "Marching Through Georgia" Syndrome

Now we come to *Gone with the Wind* which, I suppose, has to happen sooner or later with anything even remotely southern. Everybody has a favorite scene from that movie. Roy Bill kind of favors the part where the Union soldier takes a load of shot smack in the face. Roy Bill's wife, Eleanor, who was one of the few women in town who signed the ERA petition some years back, likes the scene where Melanie almost dies having Ashley's baby. She says it sums up womanhood in a nutshell, whatever that means.

Leona down at the coffee shop, who is a real man's woman, loves the scene where Rhett carries Scarlett up the stairs kicking and screaming to beat the band.

It's real revealing to ask folks about their favorite scene in *Gone with the Wind,* almost as much fun as the ink blot test. Me, I have no doubts about which scene made me the man I am today, the rather large man I am today, that is. It's that one where Scarlett is standing out in the field, all dirty and raggedy and starving, but still gorgeous.

All she can find to eat in the garden is one stringy old radish. It's hot as Hades, and it makes her sick. So Scarlett raises her fist to the sky and shouts, "As God is my witness, I'll never be hungry again."

I truly believe that those words shaped my life—and my midsection. And although I can't prove it, I suspect that Scarlett's words may have determined the eating habits of the entire southeastern United States. "I'll never be hungry again" is the *real* battle cry of Dixie, if you ask me. When people who have never been to the South first see us eat, they are likely to say that they've never seen anything like it. I'm not necessarily talking about table manners. I'm talking about volume. Having traveled a good bit myself, I have to admit they are right.

It is hard to describe how southerners eat if you've never actually observed it. The closest thing I can compare it to is the time my son made me sit down and watch a *National Geographic* television special that showed sharks in the middle of a feeding frenzy. Shucks, I've seen worse than that at the annual Ferguson family reunion.

Southerners don't eat to live or to be sociable, not really. Southerners eat with a kind of desperation, like they're going to the electric chair in the morning. In Birmingham and Charleston and Orlando and Athens, platters and bowls are passed and emptied with a speed that suggests that the diners can hear the boots of Yankee troops coming up the driveway to confiscate everything on the table and in the pantry. More than appetite is involved here. It's a matter of patriotism. Southerners feel duty bound to destroy all the supplies before they can be commandeered by the enemy.

Anybody who expects to lose any weight at all must be constantly on guard against this. Whenever we feel the onset of mealtime panic, it's helpful to repeat, "The War has been over for a very long time, and there's enough food for everybody."

I don't mean to make light of this. I'm convinced that we southerners are really, truly afraid of being hungry, just like some people are afraid of snakes or of Dan Quayle ever becoming president. Fear of hunger is what keeps us dialing Domino's Pizza and driving to the Krispy Kreme doughnut shop in the middle of the night.

There should be a name for the fear of hunger pangs, like all those other northern phobias. "Pangophobia," maybe. Even when they're so full they could bust, pangophobiacs have to take that extra catfish or slice of pecan pie. Sure, they're not hungry *now,* but they could get hungry later. Probably will. And later, all the catfish and pie will be gone because their friends and neighbors are pangophobiacs, too.

It's not all our fault. Blame it on Scarlett.

TWO

What Is Southern Food, Anyhow?

Even southerners have a hard time defining southern food anymore, particularly if they have children and live in the suburbs. My own family astounded me when I brought up the subject recently.

As so often happens, I was the last to know the depth of their ignorance about southern culture. The discovery descended on me like a swarm of gnats one warm Friday afternoon as I was dusting off my tackle box. I remarked to my son that Saturday would be a good day to go out to the lake. Perhaps we could make a day of it, I said. We could pack a lunch of potted meat, sardines, pork and beans, saltine crackers, and a six-pack of Nehis. We might as well throw in a box of Moon Pies as insurance against starvation.

My son, who operates a computer with one hand and knows more about factoring equations than I care about, stared at me blankly. "Any problems?" I asked, digging under a pile of scrap lumber in search of my favorite fishing rod.

"Yeah," he said with the eloquent politeness of a sixteen-year-old. "What's a potted meat?"

"You've never eaten potted meat?" I asked, incredulous at this gap in his education.

"Maybe in school. Is it anything like meat loaf?"

"Potted meat is potted meat. It comes in a little can like deviled ham, only it's about five times as good. Rich folks eat deviled ham on little crackers for hors d'oeuvres. People like us eat potted meat on saltine crackers while we're waiting for a big lunker to strip the gears on our fishing reel."

"Oh," he said, then wandered off to kick footballs over the power lines in hopes of attracting the attention of the teenage girl next door.

I sat down on a pile of scrap two-by-fours, feeling like weeping. My own son had probably secretly sampled beer, wine, and untold controlled substances, but his lips had never touched potted meat.

"Well, it's my own fault," I rationalized. Like so many other sons of the soil who grew up in the South in those idyllic years between Harry S. Truman and Elvis, I had undergone a certain shameful phase in my life when I attempted to modify my accent and sought to distance myself from my roots.

It was well after college that I began to appreciate my somewhat Spartan childhood when children still were expected to work around the house and be polite to their elders. Still, even nostalgic parents want their children to have it easier than they did. My own parents would never think of serving their grandchildren the kind of food I had thrived on: simple southern fare such as turnips and collards, black-eyed peas and fatback. Fried chicken was for Sunday dinner or the preacher's visit. Country-fried steak was for Saturday night.

The first fishing trip with grown-ups was a rite of passage. The first sample of sardines and potted meat on saltine crackers while sitting in a leaky wooden boat was an indescribable pleasure. It was obvious that I had neglected to give my son this same opportunity.

I brought up the subject with my wife during supper. "What's potted meat?" she asked.

I was stunned but determined to continue. "You're kidding. The next thing you'll be telling me is you don't know what chitlins or potlikker is."

My wife thought potlikker was some new street drug the kids were using. My son had heard of chitlins but had no idea what part of the animal they were.

"What about cracklins," I pleaded. "Y'all know what cracklins are, don't you?"

My wife ventured a guess. "It's something you put in corn bread. Little pieces of bacon."

Close. I shook my head and continued eating my hot dog in silence, but a wave of indigestion swept through my chest. Maybe it was too late for my wife. After all, she is a Floridian who thinks country food is garbanzo bean soup and Cuban sandwiches. Whenever I have wanted to gorge myself on the victuals of my childhood, I usually have scheduled a trip back to South Carolina where my mother and aunt still cook in iron skillets on a wood-burning stove.

I knew that only hands-on experience would rectify my family's deficiency. So I called Mama, told her we were coming, and gave her a grocery list.

We arrived the next day just before supper. I had stopped at a general store on the outskirts of town to purchase Moon Pies, Nehis, and potted meat. My daughter sniffed as we entered a kitchen redolent of chitlins and collard greens. A pone of cracklin' corn bread rested in an iron skillet in the oven, while a platter of golden fried chicken glistened on the warming apron.

My aunt served bowls of liquid from the collards with generous chunks of cracklin' bread. My wife, son, and daughter each were given small portions of chitlins and collard greens.

"That's potlikker," I said, pointing to the bowls. "The cracklins are little pieces of hot fat that are rendered to make lard. What's left are cracklins. Chitlins are the intestines from the pig. They're cleaned and boiled, and then battered and fried."

"I hope they taste better than they smell," my son said, poking at them with his fork.

"They'd have to," my wife countered, reaching for the platter of fried chicken.

By the time the meal was over, my children had tried at least one bite of everything. Later, sitting on the front porch watching the lightning bugs, my son opened a can of potted meat and ate it on saltines. My daughter tried and liked it, too. Then they ate the Moon Pies and drank the Nehis.

Feeling somewhat satisfied with myself, I stretched and remarked that in the morning we could have grits and eggs and fried fatback.

"What's a fatback?" my daughter asked.

"I'm not sure," my son answered, "but I think it's an overweight illegal alien."

THREE

Getting Started

I think it was either Confucius or Davy Crockett who said a thousand-mile journey begins with a single step. Like the doctor at the mental hospital told my cousin Elwood's wife, Alma, "Ma'am, it took him forty years to get this crazy. Don't expect us to get him back to normal in forty minutes."

They were right. Six months later Elwood was just as sane as you or me. He divorced Alma and got a job as a hairdresser at the Cut and Run Boutique. He said being married to Alma for twenty years was like being slowly pecked to death by a flock of ducks.

What does that have to do with losing weight, you say? Well, first of all, it can't be done overnight. Second, you might be like Elwood and go for years thinking the problem is one thing when it is something else. If Elwood had divorced Alma twenty years earlier, he could have saved himself a lot of money and therapy.

You see, the first thing a person does when he or she begins to gain weight is to blame it on something. Women have babies; men get desk jobs. Some blame it on big bones or their thyroids. Others say fat runs in their families.

And the list of excuses keeps growing.

Metabolism is the hot word in diets these days. All the special diet clinics advertise ways to increase your metabolism and help you burn off calories. There is something to that, of course. If you have been on and off diets for years, your body naturally is going to respond slowly each time you try to lose weight. It's kind of like the wife who made sexual overtones to her husband every night at supper and then fell asleep before he could get undressed. A fellow can fall for that only so long without becoming frustrated. That's the way your metabolism works.

I am not saying that some people are not overweight because of health problems or their thyroid glands are out of control. If you have any suspicion that you have a medical problem, for goodness sake see your doctor. Chances are, however, that you are overweight for two reasons: you eat more than you need, and you do not exercise enough to burn off what you eat.

You probably know that already. "If I just had a little more will power," you say as you reach for another Krispy Kreme doughnut, "I could get rid of these extra pounds."

Most of us dive into diets with the enthusiasm of honeymooners for the first three or four days. Then we lose interest. After all, how much water-packed tuna can you eat? Who wants tossed salad without a good drenching of Thousand Island dressing? We get bored with bland foods, and the first time we go out to eat or go home to Mama's, we go overboard.

The problem is that we set unrealistic goals. We spend twenty-five years adding an extra twenty-five pounds or so, and we want to take all of it off in two weeks. Even if it could be done, in all likelihood you would put it back on within the next six months.

That is why we have to trick ourselves into eating right. Eating right without thinking about it is the key to Sonny Bubba's Southern Fried Semi-low Calorie Diet. You don't realize you're on a diet at all. Of course, you can't have three helpings of caramel cake and homemade ice cream, and you can't devour four or five pork chops and three helpings of mashed potatoes with them, but you can eat high on the hog for a lot fewer calories.

You will not lose thirty to forty pounds in a month on the Sonny Bubba diet. I guarantee you that, unless you also are in training for the Boston Marathon. If you don't overdo it on Cheatin' Days and if you eat in moderation during the week (no second helpings unless it is green vegetables or you have been digging ditches eight hours a day), then you probably will lose five to ten pounds a year on the Sonny Bubba diet. I know that doesn't sound like much, but five years from now you will be twenty-five to fifty pounds lighter. You should be a lot healthier, too, because your cholesterol should be lower.

You have a choice. You can keep on trying the fad diets and gaining back all the weight you lose later, or you can go on the Sonny Bubba Southern Fried Semi-low Calorie Diet and lose it gradually. If you choose my way, the food tastes so good you will not even notice that you are dieting.

Don't be like Scarlett and think about it tomorrow. Take the first step today. All you have to lose are your love handles!

FOUR

What Am I Gonna Tell Mama?

How to Undereat at Your Mother's without Hurting Her Feelings

Mamas have done more to make southern men overweight than anybody except maybe Colonel Sanders. If your mama is like mine, she starts cooking at least three days before you arrive.

Her favorite line is, "It ain't much. I just haven't felt like cooking lately." Right after I hear these words, I sit down to a table sagging with platters of fried chicken, baked ham, asparagus casserole, macaroni and cheese, potato salad, rice and gravy, lima beans, green beans, stewed corn, bread and butter pickles, hot biscuits, and sliced tomatoes. Maybe a Tupperware container of deviled eggs and pineapple sandwiches, too.

I always try to be polite and sample some of everything. If Mama's feeling kind of poorly, I might even have seconds. Then she uncovers a pound cake or a cherry cobbler with an industrial size container of Cool Whip or—if she's really feeling poorly—homemade vanilla ice cream.

Of course, Mama weighs about one hundred pounds soaking wet and eats like a bird. She just wants her baby boy to eat right.

After I left home to seek my fortune and had a family of my own, I learned that southern women—and probably northern and western ones, too—equate food with love. Every mouthful of apple pie you eat is telling your mama that you really do appreciate how much she cares about you.

All that cooking was fine when men worked in the fields or built houses and dug ditches all day. Eight to ten hours in the hot sun used up most of those calories. Nowadays, the most exercise the average man gets is when the motor on the satellite dish gets stuck and he has to crank it by hand to get the football game on ESPN. We need four kinds of starch in our meals like Dom DeLouise needs another chocolate doughnut.

If your mama hasn't quit cooking enough for three field hands every time you visit, I have discovered a way for you to enjoy the visit without hurting her. First, and easiest, you can hold a Cheatin' Day in reserve for a visit to Mama's. I can't think of a better reason to use one.

Second, you can stand over the table and rave for ten minutes about how good everything looks and how you can't wait to dive in. Then you take small helpings of every-thing and spread it all out over your plate to make it look as if you have more than you really do. While you're eating, keep telling your mama how good everything tastes and how she's outdone herself with the squash casserole or the fried chicken.

Meanwhile, carefully pull off the skin on the fried chicken and put it aside for the yard dogs. If Mama notices, tell her that yard dogs have to eat, too. Eat second helpings of anything green, unless it's lime Jello-O with Cool Whip. Eat slowly, too, and be the last one to finish. When Mama brings out the chocolate cake and banana pudding, politely say that you're stuffed but will try just a sample. Do your own cutting and dipping, because mamas tend to have a heavy hand when it comes to serving food.

The third method of escaping gluttony at Mama's is to lie. Tell her your doctor has put you on a strict diet because of blood pressure and heart problems. Clutching at your chest suddenly when you're walking up the back steps does wonders to convince Mama you're not a well man.

Be careful that matters do not get out of hand, however. Not long after I started researching my diet, I had to visit my mama and my aunt. "Don't fix anything special. I'm on a diet," I said when I called. But I knew a feast would be waiting.

When I arrived, Mama had lunch ready. There was a bowl of chicken salad, sliced tomatoes, and unsalted crackers. I looked in the refrigerator for the ham. It wasn't there. I checked the oven for the fried chicken. Not there.

"We just got tired of cooking so much," Mama said, spooning a small helping of chicken salad onto a lettuce leaf. "Besides, you could stand to lose a few pounds. I don't want you dropping dead of a heart attack like George did last month."

I swallowed hard. George was my age. We had played cow pasture baseball together and had gone skinny-dipping in the creek as boys. We had lost touch after we grew up, but the news was a blow.

"George wasn't all that fat," Mama continued. "He just had a big stomach. Ellen said he drank a lot of beer and ate all the time he was watching television."

She looked at me for a minute and wiped her hands on her apron. "Now, if that chicken salad's not going to fill you up, I can always cook you some scrambled eggs and bacon."

"No, ma'am," I said, swallowing a piece of lettuce. "I believe the chicken salad will do just fine."

It's funny how statistics can make you change your habits. Especially when the statistic happens to be someone you know.

FIVE

Cheatin' Days and Sleepless Nights

If nobody cheated, Loretta Lynn and Tammy Wynette would have no songs to sing. Cheatin' in love is small potatoes compared to cheatin' on a diet. I've known women who go on diets just so they can start cheatin' after a day or two. That's why the Sonny Bubba Southern Fried Semi-low Calorie Diet has Cheatin' Days built in. They are like the Get Out of Jail free cards in Monopoly.

Here is how they work. Everyone gets one Cheatin' Day a week, no matter how little they lose during the week. You can use it on Sunday, Friday, or whenever you feel the need to eat a little more of the wrong things.

If you're sincerely trying to lose a little weight and be healthier, try to follow the guidelines for the Sonny Bubba Diet the rest of the week. No second helpings of anything, except green vegetables and salads. No snacks, except fruit. And no more than one alcoholic drink a day.

You do not *have* to use your Cheatin' Day each week, but

you cannot save it for later unless you are going on vacation or something like that. Even then, try not to use more than three Cheatin' Days in a week. You don't want to undo everything you have accomplished.

If you are successful on the diet and lose five or more pounds, then you get a bonus Cheatin' Day. Keep it for those unexpected baby showers, office parties, or family reunions that will be popping up unexpectedly. Every time you lose five pounds, you get an extra Cheatin' Day, but you can use only two Cheatin' Days a week, no matter how much weight you lose. Once you reach your weight goal, you are free to use more Cheatin' Days (so long as you maintain your weight).

For instance, let's say you lose five pounds every two weeks. If you have done that, you are entitled to make Saturday and Sunday Cheatin' Days and to eat anything in the Sonny Bubba cookbook. Just be careful not to pig out for two days, leaving you sluggish and guilty on Monday!

There is a catch. You cannot have more than one helping of dessert per meal or more than one candy bar. We're talking about a Cheatin' Day, not a Hog Wild Day.

You should think of a Cheatin' Day as a reward for your hard work, but it is important to remember that the biggest reward is when you finally slip into that size ten dress or throw away those size forty-two trousers and put on some tight jeans.

Six

Eating Out

Fear and Loathing at the Brookton All-You-Can-Eat Catfish School

Everything seems to be going fine. You have been on the Sonny Bubba diet for a month and have lost two or three pounds. You used up your Cheatin' Day early in the week when your oldest daughter had a birthday party and you overdosed on hot dogs, ice cream, and cake. Since you are not scheduled to go to Mama's for another week, you had planned to eat chicken salad and work in the yard.

On Saturday morning Merle and Beryl call to invite you to see their new vacation cabin in the mountains. "We'll drive up this afternoon, and afterwards we can swing by the Brookton All-You-Can-Eat Catfish School."

Before you can say, "No, thank you, I am on the Sonny Bubba Southern Fried Semi-low Calorie Diet," you have agreed to go.

The Brookton All-You-Can-Eat Catfish School is not your run-of-the-mill restaurant. For a mere ten dollars, you get fried catfish, fried shrimp, fried oysters, hushpuppies,

French fries, fried frog legs, fried flounder, raw oysters, cole slaw, and all the ice cream and toppings you can handle. Even Jane Fonda would find it difficult to get through the buffet line without putting on an inch or two on her hips.

"Well, this is an unusual circumstance," you say. "We'll just use next week's Cheatin' Day."

Yes, you probably could do that. Once. But what is going to happen when other friends invite you out on Tuesday to a nice Italian restaurant or the children decide they all want pizza on Friday, or a long-lost high school friend shows up and you feel obliged to eat at that expensive little French restaurant that just opened?

The temptation multiplies every time another restaurant opens, so you might as well be prepared to deal with it. The sensible thing to do, of course, is to save your Cheatin' Day for restaurants. However, not everybody wants to do that.

There are other tricks you can use when you eat out. Here are some tips I have picked up for eating light at Chinese, Italian, and French restaurants.

At a French restaurant, go for the vegetables. For an appetizer, order artichoke or asparagus vinaigrette. (I know Roy Bill doesn't eat artichokes, but what is he doing in a French restaurant in the first place? One time won't hurt him.) If they have a vegetable quiche, order that along with a bowl of soup (noncreamy, if possible) and a garden salad with one teaspoon of your favorite dressing. Ask for the dressing on the side. Then take a little of it and mix it real well with the greens. A little salad dressing will go a long way if it is mixed well.

Far too many people make the mistake of ladling on a dipper full of Thousand Island or blue cheese dressing, thus drowning their salads in calories. Too much dressing smothers the taste of the salad, too. If you are going to use too much dressing, you might as well drink it straight out of the bottle.

If you want to order the fish, ask for it seasoned without sauces. A piece of broiled sole or snapper is delicious without being drenched in Hollandaise sauce. Don't even think about the dessert tray.

Italian restaurants are a little trickier. Go easy on the Italian bread, especially if it is floating in a puddle of garlic butter. Start with a bowl of salad to fill your stomach. Use the dressing as sparingly as you did on the French salad, and ask for freshly ground pepper.

For a main dish, go for the chicken. Chicken Cacciatore is good, or try a pasta and vegetable dish. As my brother-in-law says, "This is not Mama's. You don't have to clean your plate." So even if you do order something a little heavier than you should, eat half of it and ask the waiter to put the leftovers in a doggie bag. Just don't break open the styrofoam box and eat the rest just before you go to bed. Save it for another day or another person. Or the dog.

At a Chinese restaurant there are many entrees that will not add too many calories. Begin with hot and sour soup, shrimp foo yung, and boiled rice. Drink the hot tea without sugar, or—if you must—add a little artificial sweetener. Egg drop soup is also delicious, and Moo Goo Gai Pan (which sounds like something I used to encounter in the dairy barn, but is really shrimp and chicken stir fried with Chinese vegetables) is filling. Lay off the potstickers and egg rolls unless this is a Cheatin' Day.

If you are eating with friends who are not on the Sonny Bubba Diet, feel free to sample a little of what they are having. Sample, though. Don't rake half of their serving onto your plate.

I have to admit that getting through an all-you-can-eat buffet without putting on two or three pounds is a real challenge. My brother-in-law, who has lost forty to fifty pounds on the Sonny Bubba Diet, managed it the last time we were at the Catfish School. While everyone else was piling their plates high with fried shrimp and fried oysters, he methodically peeled and ate a small helping of boiled shrimp. Then he ate a dill pickle and a generous helping of cole slaw. Next came the catfish, which he carefully ate after pushing the fried parts aside and concentrating on the flaky white meat. Finally, he ate two French fries, three fried shrimp, and daintily wiped his mouth. "I'm stuffed," he said as I squirted another dollop of cocktail sauce on my third helping of oysters.

"How did you do that?" I asked him later, while fumbling around in the medicine cabinet for the Pepto-Bismol.

"It's easy," he answered. "Eat slowly and fill up on non-fried things first. Everyone thinks he has to get his money's worth when he goes to an all-you-can-eat place. I just tell myself that the boiled shrimp would cost seven or eight dollars in a fancy restaurant and that the two pieces of catfish would be another five or six dollars. So I've already gotten what I paid for. You have to psyche yourself out of the notion that you have to take three or four helpings of everything. Eat for the taste, not the quantity. I had only two French fries and three fried shrimp, and I know what they taste like now. Another dozen would have tasted the same, and I would have ended up with indigestion."

"I see," I said, burping and swallowing the Pepto-Bismol. "I wish you had told me that before I did a swan dive into the fried oysters."

SEVEN

Moon Pie Madness

How to Beat the Late Night Hongries

Cable television is probably the worst enemy of any diet. Not too many years ago, before satellite dishes and HBO were readily available to even the most remote households, life was a lot simpler. I would come home from school or work, mess around outside until dark, eat supper, watch "Wagon Train" or "Gunsmoke," and wait for the test pattern to appear.

I never could figure out what all those lines and numbers meant, but I did know that once the "Star Spangled Banner" was finished and the first test pattern came on, it was time to go to bed. Not even the worst insomniac could stand to watch test patterns! Besides, by the time the station went off the air, I wasn't hungry yet and went to bed comfortable.

With television available at all hours of the day and night, staying on a diet these days is a real challenge, even the Sonny Bubba Diet. I mean, how can you stand to watch *Caged Women* or *Reform School Girls* at 1:00 A.M. without the benefit of a late-night or early-morning snack?

The obvious solution is to go to bed as soon as Johnny Carson comes on so you won't be tempted to make a Dagwood sandwich, but that is not always possible.

What makes it worse is that for some reason the best movies come on after midnight. I was wandering around the house one Saturday night after my wife and children had gone to bed, desperate for entertainment, when I noticed that *The Further Adventures of Tennessee Buck* was on HBO. For those of you who missed this gem when it was first released in 1988, here's the plot: David Keith is a second-rate jungle guide and Great White Hunter with a taste for women, whiskey, and good cigars. Kathy Shower, a *Playboy* Playmate of the Year, plays the role of a beauty queen married to a rich photographer who, for some unknown reason, wants to be guided into headhunter territory. Kathy is understandably upset since she thought he was taking her on a Club Med vacation.

Naturally they end up with David Keith, who is sporting a scruffy red beard and looks like he hasn't bathed in three years. His personal hygiene does not seem to bother the native women, who are busy climbing in and out of his bunk faster than Richard Petty's pit crew can change a tire.

Being an armchair traveler myself, I am always interested in the geography of distant countries. Soon I was fascinated with the movie, especially when Kathy Shower began complaining about the heat and threatened to take off her clothes any minute.

I didn't really start thinking of food until the group was captured by cannibals. When the warriors began hacking off arms and legs and throwing them in stew pots, I just had to have something to eat. I was halfway to the kitchen when they untied Kathy Shower, took off all her clothes, and began preparing her for the chief by rubbing her down with low-cholesterol oil. By the time that scene was over, I had lost interest altogether in my refrigerator.

The point is that the key to overcoming your need for a late-night snack is to make sure you watch only certain movies or videotapes designed to block any thoughts of food by making you violently ill or otherwise preoccupied.

In case you need help in choosing these films, I have made a short list. You may wish to add your own as Chevy Chase makes new films.

- *Reform School Girls.* Sybil Danning plays a sexy prison warden, but the best scene in the movie is when the macho prison matron chases and stomps a kitten one of the girls has smuggled into the sleeping quarters. If that doesn't take your mind off Moon Pies and RC, nothing will.
- Any *Jaws* movie. I didn't go to Long John Silver's, not to mention the beach, for a year or more after I saw the first one.
- *Shark's Treasure.* Cornel Wilde, good guys, bad guys, sunken treasure, and tiger sharks. This is OK to watch, unless seeing sharks in a feeding frenzy makes you hungry.
- *King Solomon's Mines* (the remake). Richard Chamberlain may have done a good job as Dr. Kildare, but he just doesn't cut it in this bomb. It is enough to put an insomniac to sleep.
- Any of the *Friday the 13th* movies.
- Any of the horror movies where teenagers go to a strange mountain camp with a lake where someone was killed.
- Any Chevy Chase movie, especially *National Lampoon's Vacation.* Check out the scene where Chevy and the family visit the poor white trash cousins, and they serve hamburger helper (without the hamburger) on buns with lots of catsup.
- *Grease.* One look at the amount of hair oil John Travolta used, and you will never touch a French fry again.
- Any John Travolta movie in which he dances.
- Any John Travolta movie in which he does not dance.

If you still have this gnawing feeling in the pit of your stomach after visiting one of these turkeys, pop some unsalted, unbuttered popcorn in one of those hot-air poppers and pop open a diet drink. Any fruit is good, too, but you probably will not want to eat anything that healthy late at night. Also, I have discovered that a V-8 cocktail is not bad, either, if I shake in a few drops of Tabasco sauce and stir with a celery stick.

The following movies are to be watched only on Cheatin' Days:

- *Tom Jones.* If you haven't seen the eating scene, you are in for a treat. I have not seen this much food consumed in so short a time since I went to the last Ferguson family reunion.
- *They're Killing the Great Chefs of Europe.* I don't need to explain this one. You'll see.
- *The Godfather.* I don't care if there is a lot of blood and violence in this movie. When the fat guy started cooking the spaghetti with Italian sausages, I was willing to join the Corleone family just for a taste.

EIGHT

The Sonny Bubba Low-impact Aerobic Workout

Why Exercising Your Hunting Dog Is Good for Your Heart

Surely every man my age has seen the Charles Atlas ads in comic books and magazines promising to turn ninety-pound weaklings into towers of strength. I almost tried the program once, but instead I ordered a barbell-by-mail course where they sent me an additional iron plate each week. I was a 130-pound weakling when I started. Six months later I was still a 130-pound weakling, but you should have seen my mailman. He went on to enter the Mr. Southeast Bodybuilder contest, finishing third.

I gave up my efforts to become Mr. Olympia shortly after seeing *Hercules Unchained* starring Steve Reeves at the

Highway 25 Drive-in in my hometown of Greenwood, South Carolina. I don't remember if it was in that movie or in the earlier one that Steve (playing Hercules, of course) was captured and each of his arms was tied to a huge, fiery stallion. The idea was that the horses would tear him into pieces, but Steve was too strong.

Back then movies did not contain the Don't Try This At Home warnings like they do today on television. We didn't have fiery stallions on our farm, but we did have some fiery pigs. Roy Bill convinced me to take some baling twine and tie each of my arms to a large shoat. By the time Roy Bill caught up with the pigs and me several minutes later, I had been dragged through two mudholes, a rockpile, and a very thick stand of blackberry brambles.

The next time I experienced anything that traumatic was when my wife cajoled me into signing up for an aerobics class at the Fitness International Club in Snellville.

I protested violently, but threats of divorce or loss of home-cooked meals will make cowards out of even the boldest man. So I soon found a pair of shorts with an elastic waistband, put on my T-shirt and tennis shoes, and dutifully walked into the fitness center.

One of the instructors asked me to fill out a form, then took me into the locker room to get my height and weight. I was slightly under six feet and weighed 206 pounds.

"Is that about the right weight for my height?" I asked.

"I'm afraid not," he said, suppressing a chuckle. "You really should be seven feet tall."

After that, a woman instructor escorted me down the hall to a large room with a red carpet and mirrors everywhere. Soon the room was filled with women wearing leotards and tights—all sizes and shapes of leotards and tights! I noticed a good-looking blonde in pink tights eyeing me, obviously impressed with my deltoids. She smiled and winked.

Then the instructor, a trim, energetic young woman, bounced onto the platform at the front of the room and began shouting orders with all the compassion of a Marine drill instructor.

First we stretched. Then we stretched some more. The other guy in the class did not seem to be having as much trouble touching his toes as I was. I felt like Raymond Burr trying to retrieve a chocolate-filled doughnut from the sidewalk. Then the instructor turned up the stereo real loud, and rock music began bouncing off the walls.

"Start jogging!" she yelled. We all jogged.

"Kick out to the front," she shouted. We all kicked out to the front.

"Kick out to the side!" she ordered. We all kicked out to the side. We did this in several variations, with a few sets of jumping jacks thrown in, for about thirty minutes.

My whole life flashed before my eyes during that time. I saw mounds of fried chicken and potato salad from countless Sunday dinners. There were dozens of pizzas and the triple fudge banana split I had eaten the previous weekend. Ignoring the beautiful bouncing body in front of me, I dreamed instead of floating in a cool pond with a can of icy cold beer.

Just when I thought I would collapse, we began to slow down and jog in place. We took our pulses (I think mine was 480 per minute), cooled down for a few minutes, then took our pulses again (I was now down to 479).

"That wasn't so bad," I mumbled to the woman next to me.

She shook her head. "We're not done yet," she answered.

"Everybody down on the floor!" the instructor shouted, and we all collapsed. "Extend your left leg and move it up and down."

We moved it up and down. And around and back behind. And up front again. I was ready to die.

"All right," she said. "Other leg."

We did leg exercises and stomach crunches and more leg raises. We also did something called a pelvic thrust, which I had seen done only by dancers at the Little Egypt Truck Stop and Motel.

"Keep those buttock muscles tight. Squeeze!" she said as some group called Mike and the Mechanics blared out "All I Need Is a Miracle." I prayed for a miracle myself. None came until nearly twenty-five minutes later when we were allowed to stand up and stretch again—and finally take a deep breath.

The young woman in pink tights turned around and smiled. "Was this your first time?" she asked.

"Yes," I gasped. "How did I do?"

"I was impressed," she said, taking off her headband.

"Really?"

"Yeah," she answered, squirting some Gatorade in her mouth. "For a fat man, you don't sweat much at all."

The point of this story is that there are hard ways to get in shape, and there are easier ways to get in shape. My diet works a lot better if you get up off the couch before you take root. Get moving. If you live in the country, taking the hunting dogs (or the children) for a walk in the woods is a perfect way to get exercise. If it is not hunting season, tell your wife you are looking for deer tracks. Shucks, just go ahead and take your wife with you! Depending on the state of your relationship, however, you might want to leave your gun at home.

Surely you have heard this numerous times by now, but walking briskly and swinging your arms vigorously for a couple of miles a day is just as effective as jogging. It's also a whole lot easier on your feet and ankles. If you have the discipline to join an aerobics class and go three times a week, fine. You will feel better and will lose weight more quickly. Whatever you do—walking, bicycling, swimming, or aerobics—do it at least three times per week.

If you want to make a game out of walking, pick up one of those pedometers at a discount sporting goods store. They hang off your belt and measure how far you have walked. You will be surprised how quickly the miles mount up.

More important, walking with your friend or spouse is a good way to get away from the stress of the household and have a few quiet moments together.

It sure beats being tied between two pigs.

NINE

Some Thoughts on Food and Sex

Will Dieting Hurt My Love Life?

The most common complaint I hear from friends who refuse to lose weight is that dieting will ruin their marriages. My friends point to Eula Sue Meadows at the Sack 'n' Pack convenience store as a prime example of a woman who gained her figure and lost her man. Her husband, Merle, was so insecure and jealous that he could not stand it when Eula Sue dieted down to a size eight from a sixteen in the Big Girl department at Ramona's Dress Barn. He finally ran off with the night shift waitress at the Little Egypt Truck Stop, a large redhead who brought a whole new meaning to the term *Rubenesque*. Calling her "Rubenesque" was like describing Moby Dick as a large minnow.

Eula Sue married Shug Lawson, who teaches karate by night and pumps out septic tanks by day. They seem perfectly happy. It seems to me that both Eula Sue and Merle are better off than they were, but just try to tell that to the husbands and wives intent on keeping their waistlines and their marriages intact.

If dieting is bad for your love life, why do all those Hollywood stars like Elizabeth Taylor and Dolly Parton go on diets? Do you honestly think that your husband would want to leave if you came home looking like Dolly Parton? And how many wives are going to walk out on a husband who trims down to where he has the body of Burt Reynolds? See what I mean? No matter how you package it, an excuse is just an excuse.

What you have to realize is that losing weight is not a magic cure-all for whatever ails you. If you're naturally ugly, you will still be ugly after you lose weight. Instead of being fat and ugly, you will be skinny and ugly. It's your choice. You may not be any happier after you lose weight. It all depends on how you feel about yourself.

On the incentive side, however, studies have proven that fat people are discriminated against in the workplace. Corporations want their executives lean and mean. Trim workers even get the breaks in blue collar jobs. Shapely waitresses get bigger tips than plump ones (assuming their personalities are pretty much the same). It may not be fair, but that is how it is.

"But won't all this low-calorie, high-protein food hurt my sex life?" you ask.

Well, as Roy Bill's wife, Eleanor, says, "Are you kidding? Roy Bill's idea of a romantic evening is taking a six-pack of beer over to the Little River trestle while he night fishes for crappie."

Southern men are notoriously unromantic after they marry. Before that, when a southern maiden is withholding her favors, he can be as charming as Rhett Butler. Jim Frank Wildman, a friend of mine, used to bring his girlfriend, Nancy, flowers every day and serenade her under her window every night. Her folks were a little irritated at first, but after a couple of weeks they got used to it. Eventually her daddy started yelling requests out the window while he was tuning his guitar. "Play 'Wildwood

Flower,'" he'd holler. Or he would say, "Do you know 'Will the Circle Be Unbroken?'" Jim Frank became quite a hit with the old man, but Nancy got fed up and started dating Johnny Bugg, who couldn't carry a tune in a bucket.

The reason the Sonny Bubba Southern Fried Semi-low Calorie Diet works so well is that if you do it right your husband will not know that both of you are on a diet. The food is real tasty, and there is enough barbecue, Brunswick stew, and fried tomatoes on the menu to keep him from going into what I call the Fatback Withdrawal syndrome.

Whenever he complains about not having cream gravy and mashed potatoes, mention the words *cholesterol, heart attack, high blood pressure,* and *stroke.* Tell him, "I want you around for a loooooonnng time, honey," or "Don't you think Roy Bill looks good since he's lost a couple of pounds!" Then reach over and pinch his love handles affectionately. By the time he realizes that he is losing weight, he will feel so much better and have so much more energy that your sex life will double. Or triple, depending on how pathetic it was before.

You see, those real strict diets that some folks try when they want to lose thirty pounds in two weeks really *will* mess up your sex life. Take Aurora and Dillon Mayes, for example. Dillon was so set on having Aurora get real skinny so she could wear one of those slinky dresses that he practically starved the woman. He left orders at Baskin-Robbins and all of the pizza places in town that Aurora was not to be served. He removed all snack foods from the house and packed the refrigerator with Perrier, carrot and celery sticks, low-fat yogurt, and water-packed tuna salad.

Aurora begged and pleaded with him to let her go to the Dairy Queen for just one Buster Bar, that she would be good the rest of the week. Dillon was a hard man, though. I guess that is why he has been alone ever since Aurora ran off with the Charles Chips man. The last anybody has heard about her, she had a route of her own outside Dahlonega.

SOME THOUGHTS ON FOOD AND SEX   35

TEN

The Sonny Bubba Diet Its Ownself

I know some people like to have everything on a diet spelled out for them: what to eat for breakfast, lunch, and dinner every day of the week. This chapter is for them. Everybody else is on his or her own.

The point is to eat sensibly from the recipes and to try to eat as many vegetables and as little meat as possible. Just because barbecue and Brunswick stew are on the diet does not mean that you have to eat three or four helpings of them.

Beverages are left up to you, with the exception of breakfast. Remember not to use sugar in your tea or coffee; use artificial sweetener, or drink it plain. As a southerner, I know you were raised on sweetened iced tea, but all that sugar is not good for you. Try using artificial sweetener, or cut the amount of sugar gradually each day until you get accustomed to the taste. Dropping a sprig of fresh mint or lemon in the glass helps, too.

Good luck. And don't forget to exercise, even if you only walk your dog.

WEEK ONE: Day One

Breakfast
  1 oat bran muffin
  ½ cantaloupe
  Black coffee or other diet beverage

Lunch
  1 bowl of Charlene's Chicken Brunswick Stew
  1 slice of white or whole wheat bread
  All the tossed salad and tomatoes you want *(sprinkled with Balsamic vinegar or 1 tablespoon of low-calorie dressing)*

Dinner
  Rhonda's Roast Chicken with Tarragon *(all you want)*
  Fresh green beans, steamed *(all you want)*
  Corn on the cob *(two ears)*
  Waldorf salad *(one bowl)*

Day Two

Breakfast
  1 poached egg
  1 bowl grits *(with ½ pat of margarine and 2 tablespoons of grated sharp cheddar cheese)*
  1 piece of dry toast *(or put your margarine on this and not in the grits)*
  1 8-ounce glass of orange juice
  Black coffee or diet beverage

Lunch
  1 bologna sandwich with a slice of Vidalia onion, lettuce, and mustard
  1 bowl of Tommy Lee's Tomato Soup
  1 apple

Dinner
    Tommy Lee's Turkey Hash *(no more than two helpings)*
    Sliced home-grown tomatoes *(all you want)*
    Cucumbers and Vidalia onions marinated in Balsamic
        vinegar
    Fresh fruit of any kind, or fruit canned in its own juice
        (one cup)

Day Three

Breakfast
    Cereal and skim milk
    ½ banana
    Black coffee, tea, or diet beverage

Lunch
    Barbecue sandwich *(pork, beef, or chicken)*
    My Mama's First Cousin's Sister-in-Law's Coleslaw *(one
        helping)*
    1 apple, orange, or handful of grapes

Dinner
    Renee's Red Beans and Rice
    Lettuce and tomato salad *(1 tablespoon of low-fat mayon-
        naise and Balsamic vinegar dressing and all the
        salad you want)*
    Corn muffins *(two)*
    SueLee's Strawberry Jello Delight

Day Four

Breakfast
    Hot oatmeal with raisins or blueberries
    ½ grapefruit
    Black coffee or unsweetened beverage

Lunch
   Bubba's Pita Bread Veggie Sandwich
   Fruit salad, using apple, banana, and unsweetened
      pineapple *(one cup)*

Dinner
   Rhonda's Roman Chicken Breasts *(one helping)*
   Zucchini and yellow squash steamed with Vidalia
      onions *(two servings)*
   1 piece French bread
   Mixed green salad *(all you want, with low-calorie dress-
      ing)*
   Any fruit

Day Five

Breakfast
   1 piece of cheese toast
   1 large slice of watermelon or other melon
   Black coffee or other nonfattening beverage

Lunch
   Charlene's Chicken Chili *(one good scoop)*
   Lettuce and sliced home-grown tomato *(no dressing, but
      all you want to eat)*
   6 low-sodium saltine or round crackers
   1 apple

Dinner
   Catfish à la Charles *(one serving)*
   Bubba's Broccoli *(all you want)*
   Fred's Red Rice *(all you want)*
   Brown Betty Lou *(one serving)*

Day Six

Breakfast
Scrambled eggs *(two)*
1 bowl of grits *(½ pat of margarine)*
2 pieces of dry toast
½ grapefruit
Black coffee or other unsweetened beverage

Lunch
Fried green tomatoes *(two servings, maximum)*
Corn on the cob *(two)*
Steamed green beans *(all you want)*
Stewed yellow squash *(two helpings)*
Corn muffins *(two)*

Dinner
Freddie Jean's Shrimp and Beer *(two servings)*
Mama's First Cousin's Sister-in-Law's Coleslaw *(help yourself)*
Polly's Potato Patties *(two)*
Corinne's Corn Muffins *(two)*
Any fruit salad for dessert

Day Seven

This is a Cheatin' Day, so go through the recipes and find something that you like. Miss Eula's posthumous Pot Roast is good, as are any of the other meat dishes. Just be sure to fill up on green vegetables as much as possible before plunging into the good stuff.

WEEK TWO

Repeat the breakfast menus of week one in any order.

Day One

Lunch
    Sara LouAnn's Shrimp Salad *(one large serving)*
    Lettuce *(all you want)*
    6 low-salt crackers
    1 apple

Dinner
    Diet Coca-Cola Chicken *(two servings)*
    Brown rice *(two servings)*
    Bubba's Brussels Sprouts *(all you want)*

Day Two

Lunch
    1 peanut butter and banana sandwich *(slice the bananas crossways or longways, depending on how you were raised)*
    1 glass skim milk

Dinner
    Sonny's Salmon Cakes *(two servings)*
    Grits *(one bowl, ½ pat butter, sprinkle of cheese)*
    My Mama's First Cousin's Sister-in-Law's Coleslaw *(as much as you want)*
    Corn muffins *(two)*

Day Three

Lunch
    Charlene's Chicken Brunswick Stew *(one large bowl)*
    Lettuce and tomato salad *(with low-calorie dressing)*
    2 slices of white bread
    Slice of melon

Dinner
    Sonny Bubba's Shrimp Creole *(two servings)*
    White rice *(two servings)*
    1 slice of lightly buttered French bread with sprinkle of
        garlic salt
    Fruit salad *(made with apple, unsweetened pineapple,
        raisins, and 1 tablespoon of plain lowfat yogurt)*

Day Four

Lunch
    SueLee's Spinach Lasagna *(one large helping)*
    Tossed salad *(all you want with low-calorie dressing)*
    1 banana

Dinner
    John Thomas's Hoppin' John
    Uptown Upscale Collards
    Slice of Vidalia onion
    Corn bread

Day Five

Lunch
    Cold turkey sandwich with lettuce and tomato
    1 package of corn chips
    Bowl of Tommy Lee's Tomato Soup

Dinner
  Zelma's Zucchini Pie *(two servings)*
  Oralee's Okra Fritters *(two servings)*
  Corn on the cob *(two)*

Day Six

Lunch
  Renee's Spicy Shrimp and Pasta *(two helpings)*
  1 slice French bread *(lightly buttered and sprinkled with
    garlic salt)*
  Tossed salad with Balsamic vinegar *(all you want)*

Dinner
  Terri's Oriental Broiled Steak *(two servings)*
  Bubba's Baked Vidalia Onion *(two)*
  Long grain wild rice *(two servings)*
  Any fruit Jello-O dessert *(artificially sweetened with just
    one tablespoon of whipped topping)*

Day Seven

It's a Cheatin' Day again. So break out the French toast and
maple syrup.

After the second week, make up your own diet by substitut-
ing for the items on the two weeks' diet. If a fried dish is
listed, you can substitute another fried dish. If a poultry
dish is listed, use another poultry dish. Vary what you eat
as much as possible, but try not to have two fried foods on
the same day (and especially at the same meal, unless it's
a Cheatin' Day). Above all, use moderation. The key is to
eat anything you want as long as you do it in moderation.
  Other tips: remove chicken skin before eating fried or
even baked chicken; use no more than one tablespoon of
salad dressing and mix well with your salad.

If you are at a fast-food restaurant and you don't want a salad, remove one of the pieces of bread from the hamburger and eat it like an open-faced sandwich.

Calories add up faster than you may think. Why waste three hundred calories on two extra tablespoons of salad dressing when you can eat a cup of frozen yogurt or ice cream? If you know you are going to be eating a big meal later in the week, or if you know there is going to be a holiday party, begin cutting down *before* it, not after. The same is true for vacations. Eat less before the vacation, and then you can enjoy yourself even more, knowing that you have just dropped a couple of extra pounds.

PART TWO:

Sonny Bubba's Favorite Recipes

Soups, Sandwiches, Breads, & Snacks

Roy Bill told me something one time that I never forgot. The richer folks are, the less food they serve at parties. I thought he was kidding until I got on some ritzy party guest list by mistake (I guess they thought I was related to Sarah Ferguson, that plump red-headed girl who married Prince Andrew) and went to a party in the swank part of Atlanta where the lawns are the size of two football fields and the houses all have polished wood floors with Oriental rugs.

My wife was out of town, so I asked Roy Bill if he wanted to go with me. He said he would, but he wanted to stop and get two chili dogs and some onion rings at the Varsity.

"They're gonna have food at the party," I said, watching Roy Bill douse his dogs with catsup.

"Wanna bet?" he said.

He was right. There was plenty of whiskey and wine, but all they had to eat were little slices of cucumbers rolled up with a toothpick and a dab of cream cheese and little thimblefuls of peanuts. I was out on the lawn with Roy Bill when the hostess saw us and came over.

"Enjoying the view?" she asked, trying to figure out how on earth two men wearing Caterpillar caps had gotten invited to her party.

"Yes'sum," Roy Bill said, wiping his mouth on the back of his hand, "but I sure would hate to cut all this grass."

We didn't get invited to any more fancy parties after that, but it's just as well. Jolene and Bartow always have a real good New Year's Eve party with lots of potato chips and little sandwiches and crackers. Included are some of their recipes.

Tommy Lee's Tomato Soup

4 servings

Every summer Tommy Lee goes a little crazy when he plants his garden. Last year he planted 114 tomato plants, and his wife Ruby moved out after she had canned 200 jars of stewed tomatoes, tomato sauce, tomato catsup, and tomato juice. This soup is real good with tomatoes that have gotten a little too ripe for back porch sandwiches.

    1 small onion
    1 tablespoon low-calorie margarine
    5 large homegrown tomatoes, red ripe
    ¼ teaspoon baking soda
      Lite salt
      Black pepper, freshly ground
    1 cup milk
    1 tablespoon finely chopped fresh dill
      Lowfat sour cream

Sauté the onion in the margarine until transparent. Then add the tomatoes, baking soda, a dash of salt, and a dash of pepper. (You can always put in more later to suit your taste.) Cook for 15 minutes or until the tomato mixture is thickened. Remove from heat and stir in the milk. (If it's a Cheatin' Day, you might want to use heavy cream. Go ahead, it's your funeral.) Put back on medium heat and stir well for 5 minutes or until the soup is good and hot. Garnish each bowl of soup with low-fat sour cream and a pinch of dill if you really want to get fancy.

Sonny Bubba's Squash and Corn Soup

6 to 8 servings

The ingredients below are for the broth. You might want to make enough of this to freeze and use whenever you want to make soup.

- **2 onions, finely chopped**
- **2 carrots, finely chopped**
- **1 leek, finely chopped**
- **2 quarts water**
- **2 cups finely chopped celery**
- **1 bay leaf**
- **Lite salt to taste**

Put all the ingredients into a soup pot and simmer for 2 to 3 hours. Strain the broth and throw the vegetables into your compost pile.

Below is what you need for the Squash and Corn Soup:

- **5 cups of the broth you just made**
- **2 yellow summer squash cut into slices**
- **1 leek, sliced**
- **1 garlic clove, crushed**
- **1 bell pepper, cut into strips**
- **1 teaspoon ginger**
- **Dash Lite salt**
- **2 ears freshly picked corn**

Put everything but the corn in a large saucepan and bring to a boil. Reduce heat and simmer for 1 hour. Now add the corn, which you should have cut off the cob as carefully as possible to keep the kernels large.

Simmer for another 15 minutes and taste to see if you need to add any more seasonings.

Lars' Oxtail Soup

10 to 12 servings

What's a recipe like this doing in a Southern cookbook? I don't know. I kinda like the soup myself, and Lars insists he comes from southern Norway. This is real good to take for lunch on those cold days when you have to scrape the ice off your truck's windshield before you can go to work.

2 pounds oxtails
4 onions, chopped
4 carrots, chopped
4 potatoes, chopped
1 bay leaf
1 garlic clove, crushed
1 cup red wine
3 quarts water
  Lite salt to taste
1 tablespoon fresh pepper

The day before you want to cook this soup, you need to cook the oxtails. Put the oxtails in water with 2 chopped onions, a bay leaf, and 1 of the chopped carrots and simmer in large stock pot for at least two hours. Remove from heat, let cool, remove the meat from the bones, and put the broth and meat in the refrigerator to chill overnight.

The next day, take the broth out of the refrigerator and scrape the fat off the top. Put the broth and oxtails in a heavy saucepan and add the carrots, onions, potatoes, and garlic. Bring to a boil, reduce the heat, add the wine, and simmer until the vegetables are cooked. This is a meal in itself, and is good with hard French bread, corn muffins, or just plain old enriched white bread.

Bubba's Tomato Sandwich

1 serving

A few years ago there was a country song about two things that money won't buy: true love and home-grown tomatoes. I suppose that's true. I've come closer to buying the first than I have the second. Everybody who has a little garden or a patio should try growing their own tomatoes. If you can't, make friends with somebody who does.

When I was a boy, I always knew when the first tomatoes were ripe. My daddy would carry a loaf of white bread out to the back porch along with a couple of tomatoes, the salt and pepper shakers, and a jar of Miracle Whip. He never could teach me how to fit crown moulding, but he did a good job of showing me how to make a tomato sandwich.

I still like white bread with my tomatoes and barbecue, but it won't hurt much if you use whole wheat.

Low-calorie mayonnaise
1 **tomato**
Pepper
Lite salt

Spread the mayonnaise on both slices of bread and slice the tomato into about ⅜-inch thick slices (or a little thicker, depending on your taste). Kind of layer the slices on there, two or three at once, and sprinkle liberally with pepper and a dash of Lite salt. Press the other slice of bread down over them. Now lean out over the porch rail (or the deck rail if you live in the suburbs), and start eating.

There is only one thing that will make these sandwiches better, and that's if you can get somebody to peel the tomatoes for you. That's a touchy subject in a lot of southern families. It seems that everybody is divided up into the pro-peeled tomato camp or the non-peeled tomato camp. Every time there's a family reunion, there's a squabble over who gets to slice the tomatoes. I know the peeling is supposed to be good for you, but you try eating a peeled tomato sandwich and see how much better it is.

Bubba's Pita Bread Veggie Sandwich

1 serving

Lunches were always a problem for me, especially when I was still laboring in the construction business. One summer I was working with a fellow named Yancey who always opened up his lunchbox with everyone else and took out his thermos and two sandwiches. He would eagerly rip open the sandwich bag, lift up the bread, and peek inside. Then his face would fall, and he'd bite into the sandwich like it was another unpleasant duty.

Yancey never complained, though, until near the end of August when he threw down one of the sandwiches in disgust and said, "Cheese sandwiches. Cheese sandwiches. That's all I ever get. Cheese sandwiches!"

"Why don't you tell your wife to fix you something else?" I asked innocently.

"Oh, I ain't married," Yancey said. "I fix my own lunch."

If you're in Yancey's shoes, and I hope for your sake you're not, you probably get tired of the same kind of ham and turkey and bologna sandwiches every day. Well, I have the solution: pita bread sandwiches.

The only problem is you really have to be careful when you go into a grocery store in a small town and ask for something exotic. One poor clerk in Snellville turned red as a beet when I asked him if he could show me where the kiwi fruit was. Another time I had hunted all over the Winn-Dixie trying to find some pita bread, when this cute female employee asked if she could help me find anything. I thought about it for a long time before I told her I was looking for the Little Debbie Oatmeal Cream Pies.

Lately, however, even Snellville has started stocking pita bread and kiwi fruit, also mangoes and other things you used to have to drive all the way to Atlanta to get. This pita bread sandwich with veggies is a great lunch for right after a Cheatin' Day when you feel kind of bloated.

1 piece pita pocket bread
1 or 2 slices red ripe tomato
Alfalfa sprouts
Shredded lettuce
Shredded cheese
Low-fat mayonnaise or salad dressing

Slice pita bread in half. See, there's a little pocket in both of them. Now put in a slice or two of red ripe, homegrown tomatoes, some alfalfa sprouts (they're good, I don't care what your cousin Elbert says), some shredded lettuce, a few pinches of shredded cheese, and some low-fat mayonnaise or salad dressing. Oh, I guess I shoulda told you to put that on the inside of the pocket before you put all that other stuff in there. Never mind, you'll know what to do when you get ready to make the other half.

If you really need to have some kind of meat or just want to try something different on another day, put in some smoked turkey with the tomato and lettuce, or even a slice of beef bologna.

Bubba's Vidalia Onion Sandwich

1 serving

You get the feeling that I like Vidalia onions? I do. If you can't find Vidalias where you live, you can substitute with any sweet onion.

2 slices whole wheat bread
Mustard
1 Vidalia onion

Spread bread with mustard, either the ordinary kind or Grey Poupon, depending on your taste. Slice the onion into slices about ¼-inch thick, and put 2 or 3 slices between the bread. Now eat.

You want something else? Corned beef is a good addition, and so is peanut butter. Leave off the mustard if you add the peanut butter.

Corinne's Corn Muffins

12 muffins

You can make this recipe in a skillet, too. If you put it in paper muffin cups, you will not need to add extra grease for the frying pan.

   1 cup cornmeal
   1 cup all-purpose flour
   1 tablespoon baking powder
   1 teaspoon salt
   1 egg
   1 cup buttermilk
   ¼ cup cholesterol-free margarine

Preheat oven to 400 degrees. Mix the cornmeal, flour, baking powder, and salt. In a separate bowl beat the egg with the milk and melted margarine. Stir the mixture into the cornmeal and flour until well-blended. Spoon into muffin cups, filling them about ⅔ full. Bake for 20 minutes or until lightly browned.

Crackling Corn Bread

6 servings

If you just had your cholesterol level checked, and it's too low, *and* you're simply so thin your clothes just hang off you, or it's a Cheatin' Day and you've had a really bad week on the job, you might want to cook some crackling corn bread.

Prepare the batter like you would for regular cornbread, only add a cup of cracklings. Cracklings are the crispy pieces of hog fat that are left after all the lard has been stewed out. You can find them in the meat section of fine grocery stores everywhere.

Mix cracklings with cornbread batter and spoon into a lightly oiled cast iron skillet and bake in an oven pre-heated to 400 degrees for 20 minutes or until the cornbread is lightly browned.

You won't need any butter for this. Just get a bowl of greens or black-eyed peas, a large slice of Vidalia onion, and a chunk of crackling bread, and that's your meal.

Bartow's Bologna Rolls

50 appetizers

1 pound beef bologna, thinly sliced and peeled
1 8-ounce package cream cheese
1 box toothpicks

Cut the bologna into strips about an inch and a half wide. Spread 1 teaspoon of cream cheese on each strip. Roll up and fasten with a toothpick. You can do this with thin-sliced ham, too, if you're expecting relatives who only come to see you once a year or your rich aunt's in town to change her will.

Jolene's Sardine and Saltine Delites

12 appetizers

I don't know why everybody makes fun of sardines and sal-tines. Half the fishermen in the South would have starved to death if it hadn't been for this hearty snack.

  1 3¾-ounce can sardines, drained on paper towel
  Low-salt or No-salt crackers
  Mustard in a squeeze bottle

Cut each sardine into bite-sized portions just big enough to fit on a cracker. Squirt a dab of mustard on top. If you want to get fancy, you can do a little design. Arrange on a platter with a few sprigs of parsley.

Charlene's Cheese Straws

180 straws

What would a wedding reception be without cheese straws? Charlene likes them so much she's gotten married four times. You'd better plan on saving a Cheatin' Day for these.

  1 pound sharp Cheddar cheese
  2 sticks (1 cup) cholesterol-free margarine (of if you're
      going whole hog, 2 sticks of real butter)

    3 cups all-purpose flour
    2 teaspoons Cayenne pepper
    2 teaspoons Lite salt
    2 teaspoons baking soda
      Dash of Tabasco

Blend the cheese and margarine in a food processor, or, if you don't have one of those, grate the cheese real fine and blend with margarine in a mixing bowl. Add flour and remaining ingredients and mix well.

Preheat the oven to 300 degrees.

The easiest way to make these is to put the mixture in a cookie gun and squirt them out in whatever shapes you want. If you don't have a cookie gun, roll out the dough until it's real thin, about ⅛-inch, and cut into strips or use cookie cutters to make shapes.

Place on ungreased cookie sheets and bake for about 20 minutes or so. Remove and let cool.

Bartow's Potted Meat Appetizers

    1 small can potted meat for every two guests
      No-salt round crackers

Spread a nice amount of potted meat on each cracker and arrange on a platter. You got that, Lamar?

Jolene's Pimiento Cheese Sandwiches for Company

64 triangles

Jolene used to make pimiento cheese from scratch, but since she started working second shift at the sewing room, she said she just buys it at the deli. Here's a recipe for making your own, though.

- 1 pound sharp Cheddar cheese
- 1 pound Longhorn cheese
- 2 4-ounce jars pimientos
- ½ cup lowfat mayonnaise
- 1 teaspoon cayenne pepper

Grate the cheese into a large mixing bowl. Pour the juice from the pimientos into the bowl and stir well. Chop the pimientos and add. Add the lowfat mayonnaise and cayenne pepper and blend. If the mixture seems a little stiff, add some more mayonnaise or a couple of tablespoons of lemon juice and Worcestershire sauce.

To make hors d'oeuvres, trim all the crusts off 1 loaf of white bread. Spread with a good layer of pimiento cheese and place another slice of trimmed bread on top. Cut diagonally once, making a triangle. Now cut the big triangle into two little triangles and keep doing this until you fill up a platter.

Main Dishes

Charlene's Just-Before-Payday Chili

4 to 6 servings

Charlene started making this chili when she married her second husband. He was bad to spend more money than he made, so the day before payday there usually wasn't much left in the pantry to eat. This chili tastes pretty good, though, and you probably will be halfway through a bowl before you realize there is no meat in it. Charlene didn't know this was healthy when she began cooking it, she just knew it was cheap.

1 clove garlic, minced
1 tablespoon cholesterol-free oil
1 large onion, chopped
8 to 10 mushrooms, sliced
1 medium green bell pepper, chopped
Water
2 16-ounce cans kidney beans
2 16-ounce cans low-salt tomatoes, or the home-canned kind
1 stalk celery, chopped
2 tablespoons chili powder
1 teaspoon Tabasco sauce
1 teaspoon Lite salt, if desired

Sauté the garlic in the oil with the onion, mushrooms, and bell pepper over medium heat. Add a spoonful of water if needed. Dump in the beans, tomatoes (cut them into smaller pieces), celery, and seasonings into a large pan, cover it, and cook for an hour or so on low heat.

Sorta Like Lasagna

4 to 6 servings

This is what to do when you find yourself looking up Pizza Hut's number during Johnny Carson's monologue.

1 good-sized eggplant, peeled and sliced thin
2 onions, sliced thin
2 big ripe tomatoes, sliced or chopped (canned whole pear tomatoes are better than the cardboard winter kind)
   Pinch Lite salt
   Pinch pepper
   Pinch dried basil
   Pinch oregano
½ cup Prego or other jar good spaghetti sauce
   Sprinkling of Parmesan or shredded lowfat Mozzarella cheese

Grease a baking dish with vegetable or olive oil, then wipe out most of it with a paper towel. Layer the vegetables and seasonings and sauce until you run out or begin to wonder why you started this in the first place, whichever comes first.

Cover the dish with foil and put it in a 350 degree oven for about 20 minutes. During a commercial break, or when Pia Zadora comes on to talk about her baby, uncover the dish and put the cheese on top. Then bake for 25 to 30 minutes more.

With any luck at all, you will be so worn out from all the slicing and layering that by the time Sorta Like Lasagna is done, you won't feel like eating. That's all right. Just let it cool, then put it in the refrigerator. Tomorrow night's dinner is already cooked!

SueLee's Spinach Lasagna

8 servings

This is such a good substitute for meat lasagna that SueLee even takes it to Wednesday night pot-luck suppers at the Buffalo Baptist Church.

Sauce:

- 1 clove garlic, minced
- 1 large onion, chopped
- 1 tablespoon cholesterol-free oil
- 2 16-ounce cans tomatoes
- 1 6-ounce can tomato paste (use low-sodium if you can find it)
- 1 teaspoon basil
- 1 teaspoon oregano

Sauté the garlic and onions in the oil, then add the tomatoes, tomato paste, and spices. Simmer for about 1 hour until thick.

- 1 10-ounce package frozen chopped spinach
- 1 16-ounce package lasagna noodles
- 1 cup Ricotta cheese
- 1 cup low-fat cottage cheese
- 3 tablespoons grated Parmesan cheese
- ½ cup grated Cheddar cheese
- ½ cup sliced mushrooms
- 8-ounces Mozzarella cheese, part-skim

Thaw out the spinach while making the sauce. About 15 minutes before the sauce is ready, cook the lasagna noodles according to the package directions. Drain and steam the spinach in your steamer insert (If you want to use fresh spinach, you will need about 1 to 1½ pounds; wash, pick out the large stems, and steam until tender).

Mix the Ricotta, cottage, Parmesan, and Cheddar cheeses and the mushrooms. Do not use the mozzarella at this point.

Preheat the oven to 350 degrees. Using a 9 x 13-inch casserole baking dish, start with a thin layer of the tomato sauce, a layer of noodles, then ⅓ of the cheese filling, ⅓ of the spinach, and another layer of tomato sauce. Repeat and top off with noodles, tomato sauce, and the mozzarella cheese.

Bake for 45 minutes and let it stand for a while before serving. SueLee's Spinach Lasagna is even better when served warmed over.

Rosemarie's Ratatouille

8 to 10 servings

Don't ask me how to pronounce it. I just eat it. Rosemarie is a vegetarian and is always trying to find some new recipe using nothing but vegetables. Her mother says it's only fitting that she's a vegetarian since she married Ralph. I'm not saying that Ralph is a couch potato, but the only exercise Ralph gets is when he lifts the cushions on the sofa to look for corn chips he hopes the kids have dropped.

2 large eggplants
3 cloves garlic
6 large onions, sliced
6 green peppers, sliced
6 zucchini squash, sliced
6 large home-grown tomatoes, sliced
¼ cup cholesterol-free oil or pure virgin olive oil

½ cup all-purpose flour
1 teaspoon basil
1 teaspoon Lite salt
1 teaspoon freshly ground black pepper

Peel the eggplants and slice about ¼-inch thick. Fry over medium heat for about 5 minutes and drain on paper towels. Sauté the garlic cloves, onions, peppers, zucchini, and tomatoes in the oil until tender. Stir in the flour, basil, Lite salt, and black pepper, and cook for another minute.

While you are layering the eggplant slices and vegetables in a large baking dish, preheat the oven to 350 degrees. Bake for about 45 minutes.

Eaten by itself on a Diet Day (maybe with some brown rice or a chunk of cornbread), this will fill you up. It is fine as a side dish, too.

Meats

Barbecue

There are some folks who say the South never would have had any politicians if barbecue hadn't been discovered. Throwing a barbecue is a sensible, civilized way for a candidate to campaign, I think. The only pitfall is if a greenhorn politician picks the wrong fellow to cook his barbecue and it comes out burned and tasteless. The best politicians devote as much time to finding and keeping a good barbecue cook as they do to raising money.

Of course there's no guarantee everybody who shows up to eat a candidate's barbecue is going to vote for him. Former Governor Marvin Griffin of Georgia discovered that problem when he lost an election once after a string of successful barbecues.

Barbecues aren't as significant in the South anymore, since the voters have gotten more sophisticated and a lot more northerners have moved here. There are more wine and cheese parties for politicians, and one bold candidate in Atlanta actually had a quiche fund-raiser. I don't believe he won, but it was just another example of how quickly the culture is changing.

Discovering a good barbecue place is almost as difficult as finding a seedy, out-of-the way beer joint that serves ice-cold longnecks, pickled eggs and turtle stew, like Buddy's and Jack's in Anderson, S.C. There are twice as many bad barbecue restaurants as there are good ones. My rule of thumb is, if it's on an interstate highway, you'd do better to drop a haunch of wild boar in the coals of a campfire and forget about it until the next morning.

There's no reason you can't have barbecue on a diet, especially on Sonny Bubba's diet. The only thing you have to be careful of is the kind of sauce you use and the amount. Calories add up fast when you're sopping a chunk of pork in a puddle of brown sugar-sweetened sauce.

There are other books on how to cook pigs and the amount of coals to use and all that, so I'll be brief. No matter what you're cooking—hams, tenderloins, ribs, chicken or beef—go slow. The slower the better. Instead of basting the meat with a sauce while you're cooking it, try rubbing it with a mixture of paprika, garlic salt, black pepper, and red pepper.

When the meat is done, let it cool for a bit and then carefully brush on some of the Not-Too-Bad Barbecue Sauce (see the recipe that follows). Don't use too much, just enough to give it a good flavor. Yes, you can eat white bread, but no more than two slices unless it's a Cheatin' Day.

If you really have to have barbecue more than once or twice a month, use chicken whenever possible. It has less fat and cooks quickly on the grill.

Not-Too-Bad-Barbecue Sauce

⅓ cup sauce

1 teaspoon margarine
1 teaspoon Crisco or other vegetable oil
1 clove garlic, finely chopped
2 tablespoons finely chopped onions
2 teaspoons vinegar
4 teaspoons catsup
1 teaspoon mild mustard
  Pinch Lite salt
  Dash hot sauce, if desired

Melt the butter and oil over very low heat. Add the garlic and onion and cook for several minutes. Add the remaining ingredients. Mix well and bring to the boiling point. Simmer a few minutes, then serve.

Many Southerners will say that this barbecue sauce is no count, sacrilegious, and maybe downright un-American. Well, Roy Bill says that skinny barbecue sauce is better than no barbecue sauce at all.

Carolina Mustard Barbecue Sauce

about 2½ cups

2 tablespoons cholesterol-free margarine
1 bottle hot mustard (medium size)
1 tablespoon Worcestershire sauce
2 tablespoons black pepper
1 tablespoon Tabasco sauce
1 onion, finely chopped
2 cups water
1 package artificial sweetener

Simmer in a saucepan for about 15 minutes, stirring until the ingredients mix well. Baste barbecue with this liberally as it cooks. This is not as likely to burn as the tomato-based barbecue sauces.

Plain Ol' Barbecue Sauce

⅓ cup vinegar
½ cup tomato sauce
1 teaspoon garlic powder
1 tablespoon black pepper
1 teaspoon molasses
1 cup water
½ teaspoon cayenne pepper
1 tablespoon catsup

Heat until the ingredients are mixed well and bubbling, then remove and use as a baste for barbecue or serve on the side when the meat is cooked.

Honey's Honey Mustard Pork Tenderloin

8 servings

I don't know whether Honey got her name because she used so much honey in her cooking, or it just worked out that way. Honey buys most of her honey from other people ever since her husband Axel tried to rob a hive of renegade bees and got stung several times on precious parts of his body. Axel was in a lot of pain for several days, but Honey was the happiest she had been since the honeymoon. She seemed real downcast after the swelling went down. Anyway, here's how she makes her pork tenderloin.

  2 pork tenderloins
  ½ teaspoon pepper
  1 teaspoon Lite salt
  ¼ teaspoon crushed dry sage
      Vegetable cooking spray
  1 teaspoon cholesterol-free oil
  ¼ cup Balsamic vinegar (that's the fancy vinegar that
          costs about as much as Tennessee sippin' whiskey
          and is almost as good)
  2 tablespoons Dijon-style mustard
  1 tablespoon honey
  1 teaspoon finely chopped fresh rosemary
      Lemon slices, if you want to be fancy

Cut off the fat from the tenderloins and rub them well with the pepper, salt, and sage. Coat a non-stick skillet with the vegetable spray and add the oil. Heat over medium-high heat until nice and hot. Add the tenderloins and cook until browned, about 10 or 12 minutes.

Place the browned tenderloins on a rack coated with the cooking spray and place the rack in a roasting pan. Then, in a small bowl combine the Balsamic vinegar, mustard, and honey and whip until blended. Brush over the tenderloins and insert a meat thermometer in the thickest part.

Bake in a 400 degree oven for about 30 minutes or until the meat thermometer says it's 160. Keep basting with the honey-vinegar mixture from time to time. Serve on a platter and garnish with the rosemary and the lemon slices.

Wanda June's Valdosta "Veal" Cutlets

6 to 8 servings

12 to 14 wafer-thin pork chops
   About 3 cups fresh bread crumbs, either homemade or
      store-bought
   Seasoned salt
   Garlic salt
   Paprika
   Pepper
 2 large eggs, beaten till frothy
   Crisco or other clear vegetable oil
   Lemon wedges and parsley (if the preacher's coming to
      dinner)

Buy a tray of wafer-thin pork chops, the whitest and leanest ones you can find. When you're ready to cook, trim the chops, cutting out the oval loin section. (Save the bones and fat for a skinny, needy friend, or for a pot of beans or greens on a Cheatin' Day. See index under Day, Cheatin'.) Combine the bread crumbs, seasoned salt, garlic salt, paprika, and pepper to taste.

Take a heavy saucer or a meat mallet or your son's baseball bat—wash it first—and pound those chops flat as a fritter. If you can't read Doug Marlette's Kudzu comic strip through them, they are not nearly flat enough. All this pounding is loud and takes some time, but it can be real therapeutic. (Wanda June says she likes to make these cutlets on Saturdays when her husband Earl has been out all night and comes rolling in around noon, with two of the tires on the Camaro flat and his pants on backwards. You can make them whenever you feel the need.)

After you have pounded as long as you can, depending on your energy level and the state of your relationship, take your cutlets and dip each one in egg, then in the crumb mixture. Leave them on a platter on the sideboard to dry out a bit and kind of settle in. (Wanda June often uses this time to go in and check on Earl and see if he can make a fist yet. If you're not Wanda June—and you should thank your lucky stars you're not—I guess you could go water the plants or feed the cats or something.)

Anyway, after about 15 minutes or so, put a couple of inches of oil in a large, heavy skillet and heat it the way you would if you were making those other pork chops, the unhealthy, greasy kind. Brown the cutlets over medium high heat, turning them carefully so as not to break up the crust. Fry the cutlets two or three at a time, removing each batch to a warm place and draining on paper towels. (Put these on top of the Kudzu comic strip.)

Lemon wedges give this dish a nice tang, and I'll guarantee you that nobody, not even your snooty cousin Velma who's been married twice and been to New York City three times, can tell you this is not veal. If *you* want to tell so that everybody at the table will know how smart and thrifty you are, that's strictly up to you.

Probably at this point, somebody will ask where the cream gravy is. This would be a nice time to start reminiscing about everybody in the county who's died of a heart attack or stroke in the last five years.

If they still won't hush up about having something to pour on the cutlets, I suppose you could go out in the kitchen and get some "Not-Too-Bad Barbecue Sauce" (see recipe).

Brunswick Stew

Brunswick stew is one of those items of controversy in the South, like barbecue and corn bread and biscuits. Everybody has his own recipe. The folks in Brunswick, Georgia, claim their recipe is the best one, but some other folks in Virginia have challenged them and every year they have a cook-off. It's kind of like the Alabama-Auburn game. Some years Auburn comes out on top, and others it's Alabama. Brunswick stew is one of those fine Southern dishes that's almost impossible to ruin. You can throw in squirrel and rabbit and pork and beef and chicken and it's still delicious. Here are a couple of representative recipes.

Charlene's Chicken Brunswick Stew

8 servings

3 tablespoons cholesterol-free margarine
1 chicken, already plucked and cut up
2 cups water
1 large onion, peeled and chopped in large pieces
2 cups canned tomatoes (1 16-ounce can)
1 packet artificial sweetener
⅓ cup white wine
1 10-ounce package fresh corn (whole kernel, not creamed)
1 10-ounce package frozen lima beans (if you've got fresh, use those)
1 cup toasted bread crumbs

Lite salt
Pepper
Tabasco sauce
Worcestershire sauce

Heat the margarine in a Dutch oven and brown the chicken lightly. Add the water, onions, tomatoes, artificial sweetener and wine. Cover and simmer for 1 hour and 15 minutes, more or less. Take the chicken out of the pot and let it cool. Take off the skin, remove the meat from the bones and tear it into small pieces. Add the remaining ingredients to the pot and bring to a boil. Reduce the heat and simmer for another half hour uncovered. Put in the chicken and cook for 10 minutes. Add salt, pepper, Tabasco sauce and Worcestershire sauce to taste.

This goes good with some hot cornbread as a main course, or for lunch with a salad on your regular diet day.

Bubba's Brunswick Stew

12 servings

1 large chicken (get it already cut up)
3 lbs. pork roast
3 large onions
4 tablespoons cholesterol-free margarine
1 cup chicken broth (low sodium)
2 16-ounce cans tomatoes
2 cups catsup
1 cup Not-Too-Bad Barbecue Sauce (See recipe, or add your own favorite sauce)
3 tablespoons black pepper

2 cups potatoes, peeled and cut in 1-inch squares
1 10-ounce package frozen lima beans
3 tablespoons Lite salt
2 tablespoons Tabasco
1 tablespoon Worcestershire sauce
1 cup whole kernel corn (or 1 10-ounce package frozen)

You need to stew your chicken (or cook it in a pressure cooker) until it falls off the bones. Remove the skin and bones and chop the chicken meat real good. Cook your pork roast in the pressure cooker, too, or in a regular pot until tender. Remove from the heat, let cool, and finely chop.

If you really want to make a good Brunswick stew, barbecue the pork roast outside or go by a barbecue restaurant that you know serves good meat and buy 3 pounds of barbecued pork, chopped.

In a large, heavy stewpot, sauté the chopped onions in the margarine over medium heat, or, if you want to cut a few calories, cook in the chicken broth and leave out the margarine. I always put it in and just eat a little less of the stew. Add the rest of the broth and bring to a boil. Now add the chopped chicken and chopped pork, the tomatoes, catsup, barbecue sauce and pepper. Cook over medium to medium high heat until mixture comes to a boil, then reduce heat and simmer, stirring frequently. Cook for two hours, then add the potatoes, lima beans, Lite salt, Tabasco, and Worcestershire sauce. Cook for another hour and add the corn. Cook for another 15 minutes, taste to see if you need to add Lite salt and pepper, and serve hot. This can be refrigerated or frozen in individual containers and heated in the microwave for lunches.

This ought to serve 12 unless some of Lamar's family is coming over.

Miss Mona's Meat Loaf

6 servings

Miss Mona used to be the chief cook at the elementary school lunchroom. I know that was a long time ago, but I still can remember her meat loaf vividly. It was the only thing on the menu worth eating besides the hot dogs.

1½ **pounds ground beef**
½ **pound seasoned pork sausage**
1 **egg, beaten**
1 **small onion, finely chopped**
1 **cup soft bread crumbs**
¼ **cup oatmeal**
½ **cup tomato sauce**
1 **teaspoon Worcestershire sauce**
⅓ **cup milk**
   Lite salt
   Pepper

Mix all of the ingredients together. Actually, if you wash your hands real good after playing with the cat, you can mix this a lot better by squishing the mixture between your fingers. Add more milk if you think it needs more liquid. Place in a loaf pan and bake in a 375 degree oven for one hour. If you like, about 15 minutes before the meat loaf is done, spoon some tomato sauce over the top.

Serve with mashed potatoes and English peas on Cheatin' Days, or slice the leftover portion thin for lunch.

SueLee's Stuffed Cabbage with Lamb

10 servings

If you have a hard time getting ground lamb, ground beef will do fine.

        1 cabbage
        2 quarts boiling water
        1 teaspoon Lite salt

For stuffing:
        1 pound ground lamb or beef
        ¼ cup water
        1 medium onion, finely chopped
        1 cup soft bread crumbs
        1 egg, beaten
        1 teaspoon lemon juice
        1 teaspoon Lite salt
        1 teaspoon pepper

For sauce:
        1 bay leaf
        1 clove garlic, minced
        2 cups tomato sauce
        1 teaspoon nutmeg
        1 package artificial sweetener

Boil the cabbage in salted water for 5 minutes or until the leaves are looser. Drain and hold under cold water. Cut out the core, pull off the outer leaves, and save the rest of cabbage to cook later. Cut off the big stems in the cabbage leaves and spread the leaves out flat. Mix the ingredients for the stuffing and put a heaping spoonful on the center of each cabbage leaf. Roll up and fasten with a toothpick. Place all of the rolls in a Dutch oven or casserole. Mix the bay leaf, garlic, tomato sauce, nutmeg, and sweetener, pour over the rolls and cover. Bake for 1 hour at 350 degrees, then uncover and bake for another ½ hour or longer if needed.

Bubba's Skillet Beef for Bachelors

4 to 6 servings

This is an easy meal to make for bachelors or for husbands whose wives are out of town. Waymon and Roy Bill never cook when their wives are out of town, so this doesn't apply to them.

1 pound lean ground beef
1 medium onion, chopped
½ green bell pepper, chopped
1 teaspoon Worcestershire sauce
½ bottle chili sauce (6 ounces)
1 16-ounce can tomatoes
½ teaspoon pepper
1½ cups water
¾ cup barley (or potatoes, if you don't have barley)

Cook the meat, onions, and bell pepper in a skillet until brown, then drain off the fat. Add the other ingredients and bring to a boil. Simmer over medium heat, covered, for 1 hour. This will make enough to last for three or four days, if you're dining alone.

Stuffed Peppers

3 stuffed peppers

Where I grew up in South Carolina, bell peppers were called bullnose peppers, for obvious reasons. They can be pickled, eaten raw, mixed with salads, stir-fried with shrimp and chicken, and stuffed. These stuffed peppers sound sinful, but they're only 160 calories apiece.

    3 large green bell peppers, cleaned and seeded
    ½ cup cooked rice
    4 ounces lean hamburger meat
      Lite salt and pepper
      Dash garlic salt
    1 tablespoon tomato sauce

Brown the hamburger meat and drain well. Mix the meat, rice, pepper, salt and garlic salt and moisten with tomato sauce. Stuff the peppers with the mixture and place in a casserole dish with about ¼ inch of hot water. Bake in a 375 degree oven for about 20 minutes or until the peppers are cooked.

My Brother-in-Law's Beef Burgundy

6 servings

My brother-in-law learned to cook when he was laid off at the mill in between deer season and turkey season. He said he got tired of watching Geraldo and Donahue on the TV and switched over to one of those cooking shows. Before too many weeks he was whipping up gourmet meals like Meat Loaf à la Monroe and Monroe's Chipped Beef on Toast. This Beef Burgundy is one of his better efforts. Sometimes. It all depends on how much of the Burgundy goes into the pot and how much goes into Monroe.

    1 pound boneless beef, round steak or sirloin (If you can
        get boneless short ribs, they're even better)
   10 new red potatoes, peeled and cubed
    2 tablespoons cholesterol-free margarine, softened
    ½ teaspoon Lite salt
    ½ teaspoon pepper
    1 cup little bitty pearl onions, peeled
    1 carrot, sliced
    1 clove garlic
    1 cup Burgundy or dry red wine (no, don't use any from
        that bottle that Cousin Alvin carries in his back
        pocket)
    ½ cup water (maybe a dab more)
    1 teaspoon dried marjoram (whole)
    ½ teaspoon dried thyme (whole)
    1 teaspoon beef-flavored bouillon granules
    2 cups mushroom halves (fresh, not canned)
    2 tablespoons all-purpose flour
    2 tablespoons water

Cut steak into 1-inch cubes. Put the potatoes in a medium saucepan and cover with water. Bring to boil and cook over medium-high heat until tender (about 20 minutes). Drain and mash. Add the margarine, salt, and pepper and stir well.

Coat a Dutch oven with the cooking spray and place over medium-high heat until hot. Add the beef and cook until the meat is lightly browned (don't overcook). Remove from the pan and drain on paper towels. Wipe the pan out and recoat with cooking spray. Add the onions, carrots, garlic clove and a dash of salt. Sauté for five minutes and add the steak that's been sitting over there on the paper towel. Pour in the wine, ½ cup of water, marjoram, thyme, beef bouillon granules and a dash of pepper to taste. Stir and cover, reduce the heat and simmer for 45 minutes. Add the mushrooms, cover, and cook another 45 minutes.

Now combine the flour with 2 tablespoons of water and stir into the beef mixture. Cook over medium-high heat until it comes to a boil, then cook for 1 minute longer or until thickened.

Pour the beef mixture into a 10 by 6-inch baking dish. Now, remember the potato mixture? Put it in a decorating bag with a star tip. Make a lattice design over the beef mixture (or any kind of fancy design that strikes your fancy). Broil five or six inches from the heat for about 10 minutes or until browned.

This is not bad for one of the non-Cheatin' Day meals as long as you can keep from eating more than one cupful. (That's only about 265 calories.) Fill up on a nice green salad.

Miss Eula's Posthumous Pot Roast

8 to 10 servings

I sure hope the late Miss Eula won't be mad that I tinkered with her recipe after the fact. Seems like I knew her all my life, and that she was always old. I was fond of her, and I think she liked me all right. She was on my paper route, and when I'd go to collect on cold or rainy days, she always gave me too much money. When I'd point this out—I was plump, but I was honest—she'd get all flustered and say to keep it, that it was too much trouble to go find her bifocals to count it out right. I guess if Miss Eula knew little Sonny Ferguson was all grown up and writing a diet cookbook, of all things, she'd be spinning in her grave like a top. Anyway, don't let the fact that the cook is dead put you off this dish. Miss Eula ate this at least once a week, and she lived to be 93. She always took it to the families of the bereaved, and claimed it had healing powers. Maybe it does.

    2 tablespoons vegetable oil
    3 to 4 pounds beef roast, rump, round, or center cut chuck
        with as much fat trimmed off as possible
      Kitchen Bouquet browning liquid
    1 bay leaf
      Sprig parsley
    ½ teaspoon thyme, or whatever herb you like
      Fresh ground pepper and Lite salt to taste
    1 clove garlic, minced
    1 large onion, chopped
    2 10¾-ounce cans low-sodium beef broth
    1 10¾-ounce can low-sodium cream of mushroom soup
    1 tablespoon catsup
    ½ cup red wine (not cooking wine, which is loaded with
        salt)

1 stalk celery, chopped with leaves
1 carrot, chopped
1 ripe tomato, chopped
1 carrot, cut into large chunks
3 potatoes, quartered (if it's a Cheatin' Day)
3 leeks or boiling onions

You need to make this a day before you want it, so you can refrigerate it overnight and skim all the fat off the top the next morning. Miss Eula never bothered to do this, I don't think, but she didn't have to. She was thin as a rail, and you ain't. Are you? I didn't think so.

Put about 2 tablespoons of clear vegetable oil in the bottom of a heavy pot or Dutch oven, one with a lid. Trim the roast and rub it with Kitchen Bouquet and the seasonings. Heat the oiled pan till it smokes, and brown the roast quickly on both sides. Take the roast out and put it on a platter. Turn the heat down, and sauté the garlic and onion till it's clear, but not brown. Put the roast back in and plop in everything else on top except the carrot chunks, the leeks and the potatoes. All the alcohol in the wine cooks away, so you don't have to worry about that. Miss Eula explained that she only kept wine in the house to use in her famous pot roast. Mr. Wallace, another of my paper route customers and the proud owner of the only licensed liquor store in town, once remarked that Miss Eula must eat more pot roast than any other human being in both North *and* South Carolina.

Okay, now that all of that's in the pot, put the lid on and set the stove on the lowest possible heat. Go away and do something useful, then come back in three hours and test the meat to see if it is fork-tender. Maybe it will be, and maybe it won't. If it's not, simmer it some more. Let the whole thing cool, cover it with foil or the lid, and refrigerate. Next morning, scrape all the solid fat off. You may be surprised how much there is, especially if you used chuck.

Now we come to the hard part, the part where I deliberately defy Miss Eula's instructions. She would have fixed it the night before, left all the fat in, and thickened the gravy with flour. With apologies to Eula, you and I are going to remove the roast, get out the blender or food processor, and blend the gravy in small batches. The cooked vegetables will work as a natural thickener. No, our gravy won't be as glossy as Miss Eula's, and it may turn out kind of a funny color. That shouldn't bother you. Are we here to lose weight, or find fault?

Put your roast and gravy back in the pot, and add the carrots and leeks. If you're cooking this on a Cheatin' Day, you might want to add potatoes or dumplings. Cover it all up and simmer till the vegetables are done, about 45 minutes.

If it should happen that you make Miss Eula's pot roast on a Cheatin' Day, you could put some of her drop dumplings on top.

Miss Eula's Posthumous Drop Dumplings

8 servings

Miss Eula used to say that you didn't have to chew these dumplings, they were so light. Which was a good thing in her case, since her dentures were out as often as they were in. (Come to think of it, maybe it would be good to make these after a visit to the dentist. If a root canal doesn't justify a Cheatin' Day, I don't know what does.)

- ½ cup margarine or Butter Blend
- 1 bunch fresh parsley, coarsely chopped
  Pinch Lite salt
- 1 cup all-purpose flour

1 large egg, beaten
2 tablespoons cold water, if needed

That's right, I said a WHOLE stick of margarine. If you're gonna cheat, cheat, that's my motto. Leave it out to soften a bit, then mash it up with a fork and add the parsley, salt and flour, working it like you would a pie crust. (I'm sure sorry I said that.) Work in the egg. By now, you should have a mixture that's stiff, but smooth. If it seems dry, dribble in a bit of water. Cover the bowl and refrigerate.

When it's time, heat the roast and gravy till it's simmering gently, then drop in the dumpling mixture by spoonfuls. Slap the lid on, set the timer for 20 minutes, and don't peek. (On a stormy afternoon a long time ago, I sat in Miss Eula's kitchen and watched her make these. "Don't peek!" seemed to be the big thing. She said it four or five times. Frankly, I don't know what happens if you do peek—I always had too much respect for Miss Eula to try it.)

Note: No, you can't have potatoes and dumplings both on a Cheatin' Day. How dumb do I look?

Terri's Oriental Broiled Steak

6 servings

Terri used to be plain ol' Terry with a Y until she got accepted as an airline stewardess, uh, excuse me, flight attendant. Apparently she's doing real well. She's been to Japan and Hawaii and Mobile and everywhere. Whenever she's home, she likes to whip up an exotic dish. Speaking of exotic dishes . . . no, that's another story.

1½ pounds flank steak
2 juicy oranges
2 tablespoons low-sodium soy sauce
2 tablespoons ginger
1 tablespoon honey
1 tablespoon cholesterol-free vegetable oil
1 crushed clove garlic

Take a real sharp-pronged fork and punch holes in the flank steak. Place in a glass baking dish and set aside while you mix up the other stuff. Squeeze and strain the oranges and mix the juice with the soy sauce, ginger, honey, oil and garlic. Pour this over the steak and make sure you have it coated on both sides. Now cover and put in the refrigerator overnight. You might want to flip it over when you wake up in the morning.

To cook, drain the steak and put on a broiler pan (or a charcoal grill) and broil about 6 inches from the heat for 5 minutes on each side (or until you get it burned enough to suit Roy Bill). Baste with the marinade to keep it from drying out too much. Serve on a platter cut in thin, diagonal strips. (You can also do this on a grill with those wooden sticks. Cut the marinated steak into 1 by 6-inch strips and thread onto the wooden skewers. Cook over charcoal about 5 or 6 minutes per side, basting frequently. If you want to chop up a small onion and put it in the marinade, that's fine, too. Terri won't mind.)

Poultry

Chicken, Fried and Otherwise

Fried chicken was always the main course for Sunday dinner when I was growing up, whether the preacher was coming or not. That was when frying chicken was a two-day ordeal. Mama could have gone to the Winn-Dixie and bought a couple of those cut-up chickens, but that would have been considered un-American. No, every Saturday morning she and one of my aunts would head out to the chicken pen in search of a White Leghorn or a Rhode Island Red or some other variety that looked tender enough to fry. The fastest ones usually escaped the frying pan, but eventually ended up in the stew pot with a mess of dumplings.

When the two victims were picked out, they would be hoisted by the head, slung around several times until their neck was wrung, then set loose to flutter for several minutes in a macabre death dance. Now these were the same women who whipped me with a peachtree switch for being cruel to Luther Bowick's bull. I guess I was being a little cruel, but I figured those BB pellets didn't hurt the bull nearly as much as it hurt those chickens having their necks wrung.

Anyway, after the chickens were good and dead, the women would plunge them in a pan of hot water and proceed to pluck all the feathers. The little pinfeathers that were left were singed off with a piece of newspaper that was set afire in the cookstove. Then they would be cut open, with the unedible parts (and there were darn few unedible parts) thrown to the dogs, and the liver and heart and gizzard set aside as if they were gold. The feet and necks were put in a bag to make chicken soup or chicken feet and rice during the week, and the choice parts were put in the refrigerator to await Sunday frying.

It was all very earthy and educational and all that, but I tried not to watch any more than I had to. Sometimes I think if more people were raised on farms, we'd have a lot more vegetarians.

I never did lose my taste for fried chicken, though. Unfortunately, after moving to Snellville, Georgia, I've eaten more fried chicken at the Colonel's than I have at my own house.

Don't laugh. When's the last time you actually cut up a chicken, soaked it in buttermilk, dusted the pieces with flour and salt and pepper, dropped them in hot shortening and fried them until they were golden brown and crispy on the outside and juicy and moist on the inside? Five years ago Sunday? I thought so. Fried chicken is becoming a lost art in the South, along with biscuit making. With a fast-food chicken place on almost every corner, a woman would be a fool to stand for an hour over a hot stove, brushing her hair out of her eyes with the back of her hand, and waiting for the hot grease to splatter all over her face. Well, sometimes drastic measures are called for. Nothing cheers up a man quicker than to walk into the kitchen and find his wife wearing an apron, with flour smudges on her forehead, hovering over a black iron skillet full of fried chicken. So the next time your loved one is feeling low, or is about to turn 40, 50, or 60, or is mourning the loss of his favorite bird dog, bite the pullet and surprise him. This is only good for one of his Cheatin' Days, however.

SueLee's Second Honeymoon Fried Chicken

8 servings

1 chicken, already plucked and cut up
3 cups buttermilk
1 cup all-purpose flour
   Lite salt
   Pepper

Enough cholesterol-free shortening to fill a large skillet to a depth of 1 inch or so

Soak the chicken in buttermilk overnight, if possible. Take the chicken out of the buttermilk and sprinkle with Lite salt and pepper. When the oil in the skillet is hot (test with a piece of chicken skin), dredge the chicken pieces in flour or put a little flour in a brown paper bag and drop the chicken in one piece at a time, shake well, and place carefully in the skillet. I mean carefully, too; that oil is hot. You don't want to burn your fingers and get all cranky right before your second honeymoon, do you? Cook the chicken with the skin side down first, until browned, then turn over and reduce the heat to medium low and cook slowly until the chicken is browned on both sides (about 25 or 30 minutes ought to do it). Drain on paper towels.

SueLee says if this don't put him in the mood for love, you need to jump start his battery with a cattle prod.

Rhonda's Roast Chicken with Tarragon

8 servings

1 tender 2-pound chicken
3 sprigs fresh tarragon or 1 teaspoon dried
  Lite salt
  Pepper

No, I didn't know what tarragon was the first time my wife sent me outside to get some. I thought it was one of those monsters in a Japanese horror film, the one that Godzilla fought over Tokyo.

Anyway, take half of the tarragon and put it inside the chicken. That's right, inside the chicken. Rub the chicken well with salt and pepper and sprinkle the rest of the tarragon on it. Set it in a baking dish and put it in a 475 degree oven for about 10 minutes. Then lower the heat to 350 degrees and cook for another hour. No, don't pour any water or anything in the pan.

Serve with brown and wild rice and a cup of fresh, tender green peas from the garden and your husband won't have any idea how healthy and good for him this is.

Charlene's Chicken Chili

I know Charlene has a lot of recipes in here, but her daddy used to raise chickens. Just be thankful he wasn't a goat farmer.

     4 boneless chicken breasts
     3 tablespoons vegetable oil
     2 large onions, chopped
     1 clove garlic
     1 16-ounce can kidney beans or chili beans
     1 16-ounce can tomatoes (or ripe homegrown tomatoes)
     1 large bell pepper, seeded and chopped
     1 12-ounce bottle chili sauce
    ¾ cup red wine
     1 tablespoon Worcestershire sauce
       Lite salt to taste

Brown the chicken in a skillet with 3 tablespoons of vegetable oil. Remove the chicken and place on paper towels to drain. When cool, cut into ½-inch chunks. Reduce the heat to medium and sauté the onions and garlic clove until the onions are clear. Drain the onions and place in a heavy pot with the beans, chicken, tomatoes, pepper, chili sauce, wine, Worcestershire sauce, and Lite salt. Bring to a boil, cover, and simmer for about an hour. You won't even think about beef chili after you taste this, Charlene says. Make yourself a green salad with some Balsamic vinegar dressing and you've got a meal fit for a poultry prince.

Lorena's Low-Calorie Baked Chicken

4 servings

I was real sorry when Lorena decided she needed to lose weight. She cooked the best caramel cakes and was always the one I stood next to when they made pictures at family reunions. Next to her, I looked like Don Knotts. Not any more. Lorena went on a fitness kick, joined the Grin and Gutter Bowling League and got rid of a headache she'd had for 15 years. Nobody knows where Carl went, but they think he's managing a Putt-Putt in North Georgia.

4 skinless chicken breasts
1 small onion, chopped
½ green pepper, chopped
3 mushrooms, sliced
½ teaspoon Lite salt
½ teaspoon black pepper
1 cup chicken bouillon (low sodium)

Preheat the oven to 350 degrees while you brown the chicken breasts in a non-stick frying pan sprayed with cooking oil. Not real brown, just lightly brown. Place in a baking dish with a cover and add the other ingredients except the mushrooms (Carl never did like mushrooms, but since he left Lorena puts them in everything). Cover and cook for 40 minutes, then add the mushrooms and bake for another 20 minutes uncovered.

Charlene's Chicken and Dumplings

6 servings

Yes, I do believe this is one you want to save for a Cheatin' Day.

   1 frying size chicken, cut up
   ¼ cup cholesterol-free margarine
   ¼ teaspoon Lite salt
   ¼ teaspoon black pepper
  12 strips biscuit dough (use a favorite recipe or get some of
         that refrigerated pie crust that's almost as good)
   3 boiled eggs

Put the chicken, margarine, salt, and pepper in a large pot and cover with water. Cook until tender (the meat will tear off the bone easily when you poke it with a fork). Cut the dough into strips 1 inch wide and 5 inches long. Fry the strips in a non-stick pan with a little spray if needed. (Shucks, go ahead and put in a spoonful of cholesterol-free oil if you want to. After all, this is a Cheatin' Day recipe.)
   When the strips are golden brown, place over the chicken and mash down to let the broth cover them. If necessary add a little water. Simmer, covered, for ½ hour. Serve the chicken and dumplings on a large platter, garnished with sliced boiled eggs.

Diane's Dijon Chicken

4 servings

Diane is not one of us. By that I mean she was born somewhere north of the Mason-Dixon line and talks funny. She has worked hard at fitting in ever since she married Junior (she calls him Clarence) and has learned a lot about southern cooking. Now if she could only get rid of that accent.

⅔ cup dry white wine
¾ cup water
2 tablespoons lemon juice
8 sprigs fresh thyme
1 teaspoon chicken-flavored bouillon granules
12 peppercorns
4 boneless, skinless chicken breast halves
1 tablespoon honey
2 tablespoons Dijon mustard
1 cup sliced fresh mushrooms
2 teaspoons all-purpose flour
2 tablespoons water
½ teaspoon nutmeg
1 lemon, sliced

Combine the wine, water, lemon juice, thyme, bouillon granules, and peppercorns in a large skillet and bring to a boil over medium heat. Cover, reduce the heat and simmer for 5 minutes. Put in the chicken and simmer until done (about 15 minutes). Take out the chicken and set aside to keep warm.

Strain the cooking liquid and throw away the onion, peppercorns and thyme. That's right. I said throw them away. Add the honey, mustard, mushrooms to the liquid and stir well. Bring to a boil and cook for 8 minutes. Combine the flour with 2 tablespoons of water and stir well. Add to the liquid and cook for a minute or until thickened slightly. (Keep stirring.) Pour this over the chicken, sprinkle with nutmeg, and garnish with the lemon slices.

Doreen's Chicken Breasts

4 servings

2 tablespoons lowfat margarine
3 slices whole wheat bread (the healthy kind)
2 tablespoons parsley
1 clove garlic
1 teaspoon lemon juice
4 chicken breasts, boneless and skinless
½ teaspoon Lite salt
½ teaspoon freshly ground black pepper
3 tablespoons white wine

Melt the margarine and brush the bottom of a 9-inch baking dish (or whatever size baking dish you have in that vicinity, give an inch or two) with some of the melted margarine. Put the bread and the parsley and garlic in a blender or food processor and make crumbs. Put the crumbs in a small bowl with the rest of the margarine and lemon juice. Sprinkle the chicken with Lite salt and pepper and place in the baking dish (make sure both sides of the chicken are coated with the margarine in the dish). Add the wine, bake for 5 minutes, turn the chicken, and bake for another 5 minutes. Take out of the oven, sprinkle the bread crumb mixture over each of the chicken breasts, and bake for another 10 minutes, or until the crumbs are browned and the chicken is cooked.

Diet Coca-Cola Chicken

8 servings

   1 chicken, cut up
    Lite salt
    Pepper (fresh ground, if you can afford one of them
        grinders)
  ¾ cup catsup
 1½ cups Diet Coca-Cola

Trim all the skin and visible fat off the chicken parts. Sprinkle some Lite salt and pepper on them to suit yourself. In a big, heavy skillet, warm up the catsup, dump the chicken in, and pour the Coca-Cola over the whole thing. Cover it up, cook it slow on top of the stove for about half an hour. Then take the lid off, simmer it another half hour, and it's done. I know it sounds kind of peculiar, but like E.L. said when he kissed the cow, "Don't knock it till you've tried it." Besides, anything with Coca-Cola in it or on it can't be all bad, can it?

(If you ain't crazy about the Diet Coke and want to cook this on one of your Cheatin' Days, use Coca-Cola Classic.)

Rhonda's Roman Chicken Breasts

4 servings

The closest Rhonda ever came to anything Italian was the soldier from Fort Gordon that she dated one summer. His name was Luigi and he had Roman hands, she said. She fixed this dish especially for him one Sunday, but he still moved back to Brooklyn after he got out of the Army.

> **4** chicken breasts, boneless
> Lite salt
> Pepper
> Prego or other jar good spaghetti sauce
> **2** chopped fresh tomatoes, or home-canned
> **3** fresh mushrooms, sliced
> **4** slices cheese, either skim-milk Mozzarella or Alpine
>   Lace Swiss

Buy the boneless filet of chicken breasts. Pull the skin off if Dinah Shore hasn't already done it. (Am I the only one who gets the impression that Dinah feeds all those chickens every day and personally wrings their necks and plucks them when the time comes? I guess chickens are her life since Burt Reynolds hooked up with Loni.)

Where was I? So take your chicken breasts, put them in a baking dish, season to taste, and put a couple of spoonfuls of sauce on each one. Add a couple of spoonfuls of chopped tomatoes and some of the mushrooms, lay a slice of cheese on each breast and bake them in a 350 degree oven for an hour. That's it.

Rhonda says to be perfectly honest, she got this recipe from an aunt who lives in Rome, Georgia, not from anybody in Rome, Italy. It's still good, no matter what Luigi said before he caught the plane back to Brooklyn.

Pullet Surprise

4 servings

    1 chicken, cut into quarters
      Lite salt
      Pepper
    4 tablespoons cholesterol-free margarine or oil
    1 cup fresh mushrooms (small whole ones)
    1 14-ounce can artichoke hearts
    1 10¾-ounce can low-sodium asparagus soup
    1 cup reduced calorie sour cream
  ½ cup white wine
    2 sprigs parsley, finely chopped

Rub the chicken pieces with seasonings, then brown in margarine. Put in a shallow baking dish with the mushrooms and drained artichokes. Mix the soup, sour cream and wine with the chicken drippings and pour over chicken. Bake in a 350 degree oven for 1 hour and 30 minutes, basting occasionally. Garnish with the parsley.

Tommy Lee's Turkey Hash

6 servings

You can use ground beef in this if you want, but ground turkey is better for you.

    1 large onion, chopped
    1 large green bell pepper, chopped
    1 pound ground turkey
    2 16-ounce cans home-canned or low-salt bought
        tomatoes
    2 cups uncooked macaroni or noodles
    1 tablespoon cholesterol-free oil or margarine
    1 teaspoon Lite salt
    1 teaspoon pepper
    1 teaspoon chili powder
    ½ cup water

Sauté the onion and pepper in oil and add the ground turkey. Cook until the turkey is done and add the tomatoes, macaroni or noodles, seasonings and spices, and the water. Cover and cook in a casserole dish in a preheated 350 degree oven for 30 minutes, then take off the cover and bake for another 20 minutes. You can feel your cholesterol dropping when you eat this.

Seafood

Some of my most pleasant memories are of the fishing trips I took with my Uncle Jim on Clark Hill reservoir back in the '50s when waterskiiers were still a minority. We stocked the boat with minnows, crickets, and worms for the fish, the Vienna sausages, pork and beans, sardines, saltine crackers and Pepsis for us. Uncle Jim would throw in a couple of six packs of beer just in case the motor quit on us and we were forced to live off the land for an hour or two.

We cooked everything we caught, but those were the days when folks thought cholesterol was some new laxative, so the fish were rolled in corn meal and dropped into a couple of inches of hot lard. The crispy, fried fish were served with fried hushpuppies, fried potatoes, and coleslaw dripping with mayonnaise.

Today, fish is considered one of the best foods you can eat for your health, depending on how you cook it. Try some of these recipes and see if you don't think they're almost as good as fried bluegill.

Catfish

Roy Bill, who has been hanging around Yuppies too much ever since he bought that used Volvo, asked me the other day if I knew what they called sushi in Alabama. No, I said, I didn't. "Bait," he laughed, and dished up another fried catfish.

Catfish has long been a staple in the South. We fished for catfish with cane poles when I was a boy, and my uncle set out trotlines across the coves in Little River. Some mornings he'd come in with a washtub full of catfish of varying sizes.

Catfish and Southerners have come a long way since those days. Oh, some of my friends still fish for them, but it's easier to buy the farm-raised kind. And they're a lot tastier, too. At least you know what those rascals have been eating.

How to Fry Catfish

This is definitely one of your Cheatin' Days recipes. Get a dozen or so small-to-medium-sized dressed catfish at your fish market or grocery store. Dip in beaten egg and then in a mixture of half flour and half cornmeal. Fry in a deep-fat fryer until golden brown. Drain on paper towels and serve with grits, cole slaw and hushpuppies.

Bobbie June's Blackened Catfish

4 servings

Ever since Bobbie June Whitehead went to New Orleans with the girls from the Cut and Run hairstyling salon, she has blackened everything in sight. Her husband, Wallace, said she did that before she went to New Orleans, only it was unintentional. Now she throws in some hot pepper and she's right in style.

> **4 catfish fillets**
> ¼ **cup corn oil margarine**
> ¼ **cup cholesterol-free vegetable oil**

The coating:
(You can buy a ready-mixed blackening spice at a lot of grocery stores and save yourself a bunch of trouble, but if you can't find it, here's how you make it.)

> **2 tablespoons Lite salt**
> **2 teaspoons garlic powder**
> **2 teaspoons lemon pepper (look in the spice section of the grocery store)**
> 1½ **teaspoons cayenne pepper**
> 1½ **teaspoons whole basil leaves**
> **2 tablespoons paprika**
> **1 teaspoon onion powder**
> **1 teaspoon thyme leaves**

Now, the best way to cook this is outside because it will smell up your kitchen something awful. Heat your barbecue grill real hot (gas grills are great). Put a black iron skillet on the grill (without oil) and heat it until it is very hot. Melt the margarine and mix with the oil. Combine the coating ingredients. Dip the catfish fillets in the margarine, then in the spice mix until well-covered. Fry in the hot pan a few minutes on each side. It doesn't take long.

You might want to have a couple of extra fillets on hand in case you ruin the first one or two. Have plenty of iced tea handy and serve with a green salad or cole slaw. Shucks, serve it with anything. Bobbie June won't mind.

Catfish à la Charles

4 servings

Charles was one of the boys in the neighborhood who never seemed to be interested in playing football or throwing rocks at cats. Of course his mother was afraid he'd sprain one of his fingers and not be able to practice the piano. Charles liked to cook, too, which was unusual for a boy growing up in a small Southern town in the '50s. We made fun of him at first, until we found out he cooked better than our Mamas and started going over to his house every chance we got. I have no idea where Charles is now, but he did leave me this special catfish recipe before he disappeared.

    4 cups chicken broth (canned or homemade)
    ½ cup white wine
    2 tablespoons chopped parsley
    1 sprig fresh dill
    1 teaspoon Lite salt
    3 slices lemon
    2 teaspoons white vinegar
    4 catfish fillets
    2 tablespoons corn oil margarine
    Pepper

Put all the ingredients except the catfish, butter, and pepper in a 6-quart pot and bring to a boil. Drop the catfish in the liquid and simmer covered for 8 to 10 minutes. When the fish begins to flake it is done. For goodness' sake, don't overcook. Melt the margarine, add a dash of freshly ground black pepper and brush on the fish when served.

Mullet's Baked Mullet

4 servings

I suppose Mullet got his nickname from all the mullet he ate. I don't know, and he claims he's forgotten. Here's how he fixes it:

    ½ cup pineapple juice
    ¼ cup low calorie Catalina dressing
     1 teaspoon Lite salt
     1 teaspoon lemon juice
       Dash cloves
       Dash pepper
       Dash paprika
     4 mullet fillets
    ⅔ cup grated sharp Cheddar cheese

Combine all of the ingredients except the fish and cheese in a small mixing bowl. Place the fillets in a baking dish and pour the mixture over them. Cover and place in the refrigerator to marinate for an hour, turning once after 30 minutes.

Put the fish skin side up on a greased broiler pan and broil about 5 inches away from the heat for about 4 minutes. Turn the fillets very carefully and baste well with the sauce. Broil for another four minutes or until the fish flakes easily. Now mix the cheese with some of the remaining sauce and spread evenly over the fillets, broiling until lightly browned.

Dilly's Baked Snapper with Dill Sauce

4 servings

4 snapper fillets
1 tablespoon cholesterol-free oil or margarine
2 lemons

Dilly's sauce:
1 cup plain lowfat yogurt
2 tablespoons low-calorie mayonnaise
2 teaspoons dill (use a little more if it's fresh)
Almonds (optional, but they make it look nice)

Place the fillets in a baking dish and brush lightly with oil or margarine. Squeeze lemon juice over fillets and set in refrigerator, covered, while you make Dilly's sauce.

Blend together the yogurt, mayonnaise, and dill, and refrigerate.

When you are ready to cook this, preheat the oven to 350 degrees, cover and cook the fish (without dill sauce) for 20 minutes. Pour off excess liquid and spread Dilly's sauce over the fish. Place under broiler until the sauce starts to bubble and serve with the almonds, if you like.

Sonny's Salmon Cakes

8 Cakes

1 15½-ounce can fancy salmon (or get the inexpensive
    kind and pick all the skin and bones out)
1 egg, beaten
⅓ cup milk
1 cup cracker crumbs, unsalted
1 tablespoon black pepper
1 teaspoon Tabasco sauce
1 teaspoon Worcestershire sauce
1 tablespoon mustard

Combine the salmon and egg and stir in all of the other ingredients. (Put the salmon liquid in, too.) Mix well and spoon into non-stick muffin tins sprayed with vegetable shortening. Bake in a 350 degree oven for 30 minutes. Try one and see if you don't think it's almost as good as fried salmon patties. Yeah, I know, you can't taste the grease, but just spread a little mustard or catsup on them and nobody will be able to tell the difference.

SueLee's Scalloped Oysters

4 servings

SueLee quit cooking these after her sixth child was born, but she says it's all right for you to try them. Just be careful.

        1 pint fresh oysters
        2 tablespoons finely chopped onion
        ½ cup cholesterol-free, low-calorie margarine
        ¾ cup skim milk
        1 clove garlic
        1 teaspoon lemon juice
        1 teaspoon Lite salt
        ½ teaspoon pepper
     1½ cups cracker crumbs (make your own from the butter
                kind or the saltine kind, but use the unsalted,
             if possible)
        Dash parsley

Place the oysters and oyster liquid in a baking dish and bake in a preheated 350 degree oven until the edges begin to curl. Take out and drain. Sauté the onion in the margarine until tender and add the oysters and other ingredients except for ½ cup of the cracker crumbs. Pour into a lightly-greased (with some of the cholesterol-free margarine) baking dish. Sprinkle the rest of the crumbs over the casserole and bake at 350 degrees for about 20 minutes.

Renee's Spicy Shrimp and Pasta

4 servings

Renee says her husband Milo likes this so much he's quit complaining about the snow peas. Besides, it's only about 300 calories a serving.

    8 ounces angel hair pasta
    1 small sweet red pepper (a green bell pepper that's
        turned red)
   12 snow peas (the ones you don't have to shell)
    1 tablespoon cholesterol-free margarine
    1 clove garlic
    1 tablespoon all-purpose flour
    ½ cup white wine
    ⅔ cup low-sodium chicken broth
    ½ teaspoon basil
    ½ teaspoon Lite salt
      Dash black pepper
    ¼ teaspoon Tabasco sauce
    1 pound medium shrimp, the freshest you can find,
        peeled and deveined
    1 teaspoon grated lemon rind
    1 or 2 sprigs parsley, chopped

Cook the pasta according to directions. Use spray vegetable shortening on a large skillet and heat on medium high. Cut the pepper into thin strips and cook with the snow peas, stirring frequently, until tender but crisp (3 or 4 minutes). Place in a bowl and add margarine to the skillet, turning the heat down to medium. Sauté the garlic for a minute or two, and add the flour gradually, stirring with a fork to blend in with the margarine. Add the wine a little at a time, continuing to stir until smooth. Now you can add ½ cup of chicken broth and the other ingredients except the shrimp, the lemon peel, and the parsley. Simmer until bubbling, then add the shrimp. Reduce the heat to medium low and cook covered for about 5 minutes. Add the peppers and snow peas and cook for another minute.

When everybody's ready to eat, serve this tossed with the pasta, the remaining chicken broth, lemon peel and parsley.

Sonny Bubba's Shrimp Creole

8 servings

1 small onion, chopped
½ bell pepper, chopped
1 stalk celery, chopped
1 clove garlic, crushed
1 teaspoon cholesterol-free margarine
⅓ cup low-sodium chicken broth
2 16-ounce cans tomatoes
1 teaspoon cayenne pepper
1 teaspoon black pepper
1 teaspoon Lite salt
⅓ cup chili sauce
2 pounds fresh shrimp, cleaned, deveined and deheaded

Cook the onion, green pepper, celery and garlic in the margarine (or you can leave out the margarine and sauté everything in the chicken broth) until tender. Use a large skillet, because you're going to add everything else. Add the tomatoes and all of the other ingredients except the shrimp, and simmer until thickened. Add the shrimp and cook over medium heat until the shrimp are just done (10 to 15 minutes). Don't overcook. Serve with rice and a green salad and you have a fine meal that's not too heavy.

Freddie Jean's Shrimp and Beer

10 servings

Freddie Jean's the one I told you about who found out that cholesterol was not something you put in foreign cars. She always seemed to have a few cans of beer in the refrigerator, so this seemed a natural.

5 pounds fresh shrimp, with heads removed
1 package shrimp boil seasonings
3 cans beer, lite or any kind
1 quart water

Pour the beer and water in a large pot and heat to boiling. Put in the shrimp and wait until everything comes to a boil again, then reduce the heat to low and cover. The shrimp will be ready in about 15 minutes or when they all turn pink and float to the top. Serve with a low-sodium cocktail sauce, or make your own with low-sodium diet catsup and some horseradish or Tabasco sauce and lemon juice mixed in.

Sara LouAnn's Shrimp Salad

6 servings

Sara LouAnn always wanted to be one of those hostesses who gave fancy parties. Even when she was a little girl, she'd put little bitty pieces of sardines on saltine crackers and serve them on her mother's silverplated tray. When she graduated from high school, her mama took her aside and said, "Sara LouAnn, now you need to find yourself a rich husband." Sara LouAnn followed her mama's advice, but every rich husband she found refused to leave his wife, so she finally settled for Arthur at the BantyBurger.

About five or six times a year Sara LouAnn gets the itch to be a hostess again, so she invites a bunch of us over to play poker with Arthur (he's a terrible poker player; he always grins when he's got more than a pair) and fixes some little sandwiches with the crust cut off and shrimp salad with Ritz crackers. Sara LouAnn's shrimp salad is so good you might not want to wait until a poker night to eat it.

2 pounds medium shrimp, as fresh as you can find them, shelled, headed, deveined and steamed until pink
¼ cup reduced calorie mayonnaise
¼ cup plain lowfat yogurt
1 tablespoon finely chopped fresh dill
2 tablespoons capers (that's right, capers. Look for them in the gourmet section of your local grocery store.)
Dash Lite salt
Dash pepper

Mix all of the ingredients well and serve on lettuce leaves with crackers to suit your taste. If you don't have any trouble with your cholesterol, you might try adding a couple of chopped boiled eggs to it for a change.

Game

How To Cook What They Drag In

Wild game is not inexpensive. Oh, sure, hunters like to tell their wives how much money they're saving them on the grocery bill every time they bring home some venison or quail, but if you were to figure up all of the expenses involved, you'd be astonished.

I was never a great hunter. All my male relatives are crack shots and expert trackers, but I never have been able to get the hang of it.

My Uncle George tried to make me a hunter. When I was

a kid, Uncle George took me into the woods every weekend during hunting season to stalk the feared rabbit and deadly quail.

Every trip with Uncle George was an adventure. Not only was he a good shot, he was a better liar. "Stay quiet," he'd tell me after I had sneezed or made some other sound. "We don't want to let the animals hear us. There might be a wild boar lurking in the underbrush."

Of course, Uncle George continually smoked Chesterfields as we crept along the narrow paths. "What about your cigarette smoke?" I asked innocently one day.

"They can't hear that," he said, walking ahead.

Uncle George's hunting trips always seemed to be scheduled on the coldest, wettest days possible. By noon I was ready to go home, but Uncle George insisted on walking through every swamp and down every creek. He'd backtrack six miles just to cross a swamp we missed on our first trip.

I think the difference between Uncle George and me was that Uncle George always looked like a hunter: I didn't. He would start dressing at 4 in the morning and put on long underwear, two pairs of socks, his camouflage pants and shirt, his hunting jacket with three dozen pockets, and his boots. Then he would put a pair of socks on over his boots to cushion the sound.

Next he put on makeup with more care than Boy George, smearing green and black patches of grease over his face in a camouflage pattern. Finally he would take a few sprigs of cedar and poke them in his cap.

To a sleepy boy on a cold winter morning Uncle George looked exactly like a bush.

I, on the other hand, had to wear blue jeans and brogans, a flannel shirt and an old jacket. Even with a gun, I looked nothing like a hunter.

Uncle George finally gave up on me when I became more interested in kissing girls than shooting deer. I was relieved at the time, but as I grew older and had a son of my own, I began to have second thoughts. So did my wife.

"You really need to take your son hunting," she said one

week. "Fathers and sons are supposed to do that sort of thing. It creates a bond between them."

"I guess you're right," I agreed, and walked into my son's room to pry the stereo headsets off his ears.

"You want to go hunting?" I asked over the screams of some rock star.

"No," he said, and slipped the headphones back over his ears.

I reported this to my wife, who insisted that I force him to go hunting with me and enjoy it.

"We don't have any guns or clothes," I said, thinking about the football games I would miss on television.

"I didn't know you needed special clothes for hunting," she said.

"Absolutely," I said, remembering my own makeshift hunting outfit as a teenager. "If we don't have the proper clothes, we'll be laughed out of the woods."

"Well, go buy them," she said. "You really need to start doing manly things with your son before he's grown."

Dutifully, I called Georgia Outdoors to check on hunting equipment.

"What does the well-dressed hunter need to buy?" I asked.

"It depends on the kind of hunting you want to do," the manager said.

"Oh, I guess I'll try deer hunting."

The manager reeled off a list of items starting with American Footwear Goretex boots for $89.95, sock liners for $3.25, wool socks for $5, a jacket and bib overalls for $79, a chamois shirt for $20, Goretex hat for $15.95, and a mesh safety vest for $6.95.

"Oh, yes," he added. "You'll also need a good pair of insulated underwear. The trend these days is for hunters to wear layers of clothes instead of one outfit. As the temperature rises, you take off another layer."

"Will I need anything else?" I asked.

"How about guns? Do you have a deer rifle?"

I didn't. The average price of a good Remington was about $349, plus the costs of bullets.

GAME   119

By my rough addition, I figured it would cost my son and me about $1,200 to be properly outfitted. I thanked the store manager and reported the conversation to my wife, acting very enthusiastic.

"You know," I said, thumbing through a copy of The Deer Hunter's Bible, "I can't wait to get out in the woods with my son. He's real excited, too, and wants a couple of shotguns for Christmas. We'll probably have to buy a guncase for the den."

"How much did you say all this is going to cost?" she asked, frowning.

"Oh, about twelve hundred dollars," I replied.

"I don't know if this is such a good idea," she said. "Twelve hundred dollars is a lot of money."

"I think you're absolutely right," I said, closing the book. "Besides, nothing creates a bond between fathers and sons like watching football games on TV together."

If you are married or going with somebody who is an avid hunter, chances are you already know how to cook what they drag in. If you're about to marry into a family like this, then you'd better pay close attention.

Roy Bill's Roasted Dove

Take as many doves as you've killed that day and figure on two per serving. Like so many other foods, birds are best eaten as fresh as possible, although they can be dressed and frozen for later. (Plucking and dressing are a man's work. "You killed it, you clean it," is a motto that you should have framed in needlepoint and hung in the kitchen.) Put the doves in a roasting pan on their sides with a couple of tablespoons of water. Take a half-strip of bacon and cover the breast (of the dove, silly—some cooks take these instructions so literally). Bake in a preheated oven at 475 degrees for 4 minutes, flip the doves over to the other side, and move the bacon over to the other breast. Roast for another 4 or 5 minutes. The center of the breast should be light pink. The best way to ruin a dove is to overcook it, so be careful.

Donnell's Ducks à la Orange Juice

6 to 8 servings

2 ducks, depending on how large and hungry a crowd
     you've got
2 large apples
2 medium onions
  Dash cinnamon

4 slices bacon
½ cup freshly squeezed orange juice
½ cup dry red wine
   Lite salt

Stuff the ducks with chopped up apple and onions with a sprinkle of cinnamon. Put each duck on a separate piece of heavy duty broiling foil and lay a couple of strips of bacon on each duck. Brown in a 425 degree oven for 30 minutes, then reduce the heat to 325 degrees. Put half of the orange juice and wine on each duck and seal tightly with foil. Bake for 3½ to 4 hours, depending on the size of the ducks. Do not open foil to peek in for at least 3½ hours.

Ramona's Roast Quail

4 servings

And you thought all Ramona did was run her Dress Barn. No, Ramona's success in the garment business has freed up her lazy husband Joe Ron to hunt and fish at his leisure. And Joe Ron has more leisure than you and me put together. Some wives would complain, I suppose, but you wouldn't if you saw Joe Ron. Imagine Gabby Hayes as a young man, only scruffier, and that's Joe Ron. He's a good shot, though, and brings home a variety of game for Ramona to experiment with.

4 quail, or one per person
4 slices of thin, lean bacon
1 tablespoon low-calorie margarine

⅓ cup diluted lemon juice (put about 2 tablespoons of
     water in freshly-squeezed lemon juice)
1 tablespoon Lite salt
1 tablespoon freshly ground black pepper

Clean the quail (hopefully Joe Ron has already done this,
but you can't depend on it) and wrap in bacon, holding the
strips in place with toothpicks. Use the margarine to
grease a baking pan, or spray with vegetable shortening if
you want to save a few more calories. Combine the lemon
juice, Lite salt, and pepper. Bake for 50 minutes or so in a
350 degree oven, basting with the lemon juice every chance
you get. Some people sauté a few sliced mushrooms and
serve with this. It just depends on your feelings about
mushrooms.

Willie Mae's Wild Turkey

No, this is not Wild Turkey out of a bottle. Wash and wipe
dry one freshly-killed and dressed wild turkey. Rub with
Lite salt, pepper, and tenderizer. Chop up one medium
onion and a stalk of celery and add to a package of herb or
cornbread stuffing, mixed according to directions. Add a
half-cup of chopped pecans and a pint of fresh oysters. The
dressing should be very moist. Stuff inside the cavity and
then lay three or four bacon strips across the turkey breast.
Bake covered for 2 hours and 20 minutes or more in a 325
degree oven, depending on how big a turkey you've got.
Uncover and brown for 15 to 20 minutes.

Fred's Fried Squirrel

I told you Fred likes to fry things, even those cute little furry squirrels that invade his pecan trees. Get one tender squirrel per person (don't ask me how to tell if it's tender; I guess you have to take the hunter's word for it until you bite into one of the haunches), clean and soak in salt water overnight. Cut the squirrels in half with the hind legs on one half and the front legs on the other. Sprinkle with Lite salt and freshly ground pepper. Put about an inch and a half of cholesterol-free cooking oil in a skillet and heat for frying. Put enough flour in a brown paper bag or plastic bag to coat the squirrels and shake up the pieces of squirrel until they are lightly covered with flour. Fry like chicken, about 15 minutes on one side until brown, then flip over and cook for another 5 to 10 minutes on the other side. If this is a Cheatin' Day, and I sure hope it is for your sake, pour off most of the grease and add some flour, stirring well to absorb the rest of the grease until it turns brown, then add about 3 cups of water or water mixed with milk if you want cream gravy. Simmer until it is just thick enough, and add Lite salt and pepper to taste.

Lorena's Loin of Venison Roast

It's a good thing that Lorena likes venison, because Lumas kills four or five deer every season. Lorena went hunting with him the first year they were married, but she soon quit. She said if she wanted to sit out in the cold, wet morning waiting for a bunch of animals to show up, she'd just as soon go shopping at the Flea Market and Jockey Lot. Lorena says the loin is the best part of a deer, and I guess she ought to know.

  1 deer loin
  4 strips of lean bacon
  6 whole cloves
  1 medium onion, chopped
  1 bay leaf
  1 clove garlic, crushed
  3 sprigs fresh parsley, chopped
    Lite salt
    Freshly ground black pepper

Place the loin roast on a large sheet of heavy-duty broiling aluminium foil. Lay the strips of bacon across the roast to keep it from drying out while cooking. Insert the cloves along the loin and sprinkle everything else over it. Some people like to rub in the salt and pepper and garlic before putting the bacon on top. Seal in foil and bake in a 300 degree oven for about 40 minutes per pound. Serve with anything that you'd serve with a good chunk of roast beef.

Velma's Venison Roast with Barbecue Sauce

10 to 12 servings

        1 5-pound deer roast
        1 teaspoon Lite salt
        ⅓ cup red wine
        1 clove garlic, crushed
        1 tablespoon black pepper, freshly ground
        ½ cup Not-Too-Bad Barbecue Sauce (see recipe)
        1 medium onion, chopped

Soak the roast overnight in salted water with ⅓ cup red wine. Wipe dry, rub with crushed garlic, and sprinkle with pepper. Put the roast in a roasting pan on a wire rack and baste with the barbecue sauce. Add ⅓ cup water to roasting pan with the chopped onion and bake in a 325 degree oven for 1 hour. After that, lower the heat to 275 degrees and cook for 3 more hours, basting regularly with the barbecue sauce and some of the juices in the bottom of the roasting pan.

Vegetables

Grits

The easiest way to separate Southerners from other folks is to offer them grits. A non-Southerner will stare at them like they are part of an exhibit in the county fair. Occasionally, the non-Southerner will taste a spoonful, daintily, like a sick child facing a dose of caster oil. "I don't know what the fuss is all about," they say. "Grits are tasteless."

Then they will ask for an order of hash browns—or worse, tomatoes—and eat their eggs and sausage with an order of whole wheat toast.

Of course grits are tasteless when you eat a spoonful without a speck of seasoning. You need some Lite salt, a generous helping of fresh-ground black pepper, and at least a pat of margarine. I'm not even going to mention red-eye gravy or cream gravy. It would just make you cry.

There are ways to eat grits on the Sonny Bubba Diet that will not cause you to put on an extra five pounds. I will tell you about them later, but first let me conduct a little primer on grits for those as yet uninitiated to the subject.

Grits do not grow on trees, despite what Lewis Grizzard said in his book, *Don't Sit Under The Grits Tree With Anyone Else But Me*. Grits are made from hominy, which is hard corn kernels soaked in a water and lye solution to get rid of the husks. After the hominy is dried, it is coarsely ground into grits.

You can buy grits from grist mills that stone-grind corn, or you can buy them at your favorite grocery store. Don't get the instant kind, and I don't care what your cousin Velma said about it being more convenient. Cousin Velma doesn't eat grits. If she did, she would never buy the instant kind.

The five-minute cooking grits are probably best for a busy person. Just follow the directions and cook until the grits are nice and thick (not too thick, now, and not runny, but just right). Keep them covered until you are ready to serve them, then add hot water to thin them to the right consistency. You do not have to throw a spoonful of bacon grease in them, but you can if it is a Cheatin' Day.

Add enough Lite salt to season, and sprinkle with fresh-ground black pepper. Put just enough low-calorie, cholesterol-free margarine on each serving to give it a little color, and chop up an ounce of low-fat cheese to mix in with the hot grits. A poached egg cooked soft and mixed in with grits is almost as good as one fried over-easy, and a few pieces of baked ham mixed with grits will make a fine breakfast. Remember, moderation is the key. Do not dish up a washpan full of grits and throw in a slab of ham and chunk of butter. A little grits will go a long way.

Real Fancy Grits Soufflé

6 to 8 servings

If your mama-in-law is coming over for breakfast, and you don't want to have a regular pot of white grits on the stove, try this cheese grits casserole.

- **1 cup quick grits**
- **2 cups skim milk**
- **3 cups water**
- **1 teaspoon Lite salt**
- **½ teaspoon nutmeg**
- **1½ cups grated sharp Cheddar cheese**
- **Tabasco sauce**
- **Black pepper, freshly ground**
- **6 eggs, separated**

Cook up the grits, skim milk, and water according to the directions on the package. Add Lite salt while cooking. Preheat the oven to 425 degrees.

In the meantime, grease a 2-quart soufflé dish with low-calorie, cholesterol-free margarine, and place it in the refrigerator.

When the grits are cooked, pour them into a mixing bowl and add the nutmeg, cheese, a dash of Tabasco sauce, and pepper to taste. Mix well. Let the mixture cool off a little bit, and then beat in egg yolks. Beat the egg whites until stiff, and add half to the grits mixture, beating well. Then fold in the rest of the whites. (That means, be gentle; use a rubber spatula or something like that.)

Remove the chilled soufflé dish from the refrigerator, and pour the mixture into it. If you like, sprinkle the top of the mixture with enough grated cheese to cover it. Place it in the oven and cook until done (about 25 minutes or so).

You must eat this as soon as it comes out of the oven, so

be sure the men haven't wandered off into the woods looking for deer tracks just before suppertime.

This definitely is a Cheatin' Day dish, unless you want to
have a big green salad for lunch and this for your supper.
It's almost a main dish in itself and is delicious with a bell
pepper, onion, and mushroom omelet.

Just Plain Fancy Cheese Grits

4 to 6 servings

1 cup quick grits
4 cups water
¼ cup cholesterol-free margarine
1 cup grated sharp Cheddar cheese
3 egg whites

Cook the grits and water according to the directions on the
package. When the grits are thick and flow slowly from a
spoon, add the margarine and cheese. Mix in real well and
set aside to cool. When the mixture has cooled a bit, beat
in the egg whites and pour into a casserole dish. Bake in a
350 degree oven for 30 minutes or until browned.

Bubba's Asparagus

4 to 6 servings

I was a grown man with a mortgage before I ate fresh asparagus. All my life I thought asparagus was what you got out of a can on Sunday when you were getting ready to mix it with cream of mushroom soup, Velveeta, and enough Ritz crackers to choke a small mule. While asparagus casserole with Velveeta is still one of my favorite vices, few things taste better than fresh, tender, sweet asparagus.

> 1 good-sized bunch fresh asparagus
> Lite salt
> 1 tablespoon lowfat cholesterol-free margarine

Buy a good-sized bunch of asparagus, ones with the green tips still firm and compact. Take a sharp paring knife and, beginning about an inch from the large end of the asparagus stalk, start feeling your way up the stalk. When you get to the place where the knife cuts the stalk easily, cut off that part and discard the stalky end. I know this is a waste and that some people save these stalks for asparagus soup, but I don't.

When you have gone through every stalk in this way and have washed them good, set them aside on a paper towel. Get out your big pot with the steamer insert and put about ½ inch of water in the bottom. Heat until the steam appears. Place the asparagus in the steamer and cover for about 3 or 4 minutes.

When the asparagus stalks bend just a little when you pick them up with a fork, they are ready. DO NOT OVER-COOK. If you want soggy asparagus, go buy it in a can.

Sprinkle with Lite salt, melt the margarine, and then dribble it over the asparagus. You can try this recipe with no salt or margarine. You will be surprised at how tasty it is.

Bubba's Broccoli

6 to 8 servings

This recipe is so simple even I can make it.

- **2 bunches fresh broccoli**
- **1 tablespoon lowfat cholesterol-free margarine**
- **1 tablespoon lemon juice**
- **Lite salt**

Trim about two inches off the bottom of the broccoli stalks and wash well. Take large pot with a steamer insert (if you don't have a steamer insert, you need to get one; they cost less than a ticket to a Braves game) and put about one inch of water in the bottom. Heat until steam comes up through the steamer, put the broccoli in the pot, and cover. After about 6 minutes, check to see if the stalks can be pierced with a fork.

Sometimes I cut off the flowerettes (with just enough of the tender stalks left to support them) and put them on top of the big stalks. They will cook first. You can take them out before they get overdone, which will allow the big stalks to cook a few minutes longer. For goodness sake, though, don't cook those things until they are as limp and soggy as a dishrag.

If you are eating this on a Diet Day, melt the margarine and mix it with the lemon juice before dribbling over the broccoli. Add Lite salt to taste if you must.

If you are eating this on a Cheatin' Day, go ahead and use a *little* Hollandaise sauce. Remember, it is a Cheatin' Day, not a Pig Out Day!

Bubba's Brussels Sprouts

No, I didn't know what Brussels sprouts were until I moved to Snellville. The first time somebody served me some, I thought they were cabbages that had been picked too soon. Once you get used to them, they're really pretty good.

2 cups Brussels sprouts, washed and trimmed
1½ cups boiling water
2 tablespoons lemon juice
1 teaspoon Lite salt
½ teaspoon pepper
½ teaspoon nutmeg

Boil the Brussels sprouts in a covered saucepan over medium heat until tender, about 15 to 20 minutes. Drain and sprinkle with lemon juice, salt, pepper, and nutmeg.

If it's a Cheatin' Day or you are not eating anything else very fattening, go ahead and melt a tablespoon of lowfat cholesterol-free margarine and mix with the lemon juice, salt, pepper, and nutmeg, or add ½ cup of grated Cheddar cheese over the top of the sprouts.

Willie Mae's Cabbage with Tomato and Bacon

2 servings

1 medium size cabbage
Lite salt
Pepper
½ cup tomato juice
3 slices bacon
1 tablespoon chopped parsley

Boil the cabbage until tender. Drain, chop, and add salt and pepper. Simmer the mixture in tomato juice for about 20 minutes.

Fry the bacon over medium high heat until crisp (if you have a microwave, for goodness sake, cook it in there; it's a whole lot easier and not as messy). Crumble the bacon (better wait until it cools off) over the cabbage and sprinkle with the chopped parsley just before setting it on the table.

This serves two, so if the kids are coming, simply double the recipe (depending on how many kids there are, of course).

SueLee's Stir-Fried Cabbage

4 servings

Ever since SueLee got one of those electric woks for Christmas, she's been stir-frying everything. I have to admit, some of the dishes she cooks aren't bad.

- 1 small cabbage, shredded
- 1 large green bell pepper, cut into strips
- 1 medium onion, sliced
- 2 stalks celery, sliced
- 1 large home-grown tomato, sliced
- 1 tablespoon cholesterol-free oil

Stir-fry vegetables over 350-degree heat for about 7 or 8 minutes. Cover, reduce heat, and cook for another 2 or 3 minutes, depending on how crispy you want your cabbage. This is a real good Diet Day side dish with baked chicken or anything else, for that matter.

My Mama's First Cousin's Sister-in-Law's Coleslaw

6 to 8 servings

This is much easier to make if you have a blender or food processor. If you don't have either one, you will need a fine grater, a sharp knife, lots of patience, a good supply of cuss words, and a Band-Aid or two. Right off-hand, I can't recall my Mama's first cousin's sister-in-law's first name, so I guess it would be best to leave her out of her own recipe. Sorry, sis.

1 medium head cabbage, shredded or finely chopped
1 cucumber, finely chopped
½ green pepper, finely chopped
1 large carrot, finely chopped
¼ cup green onions, thinly sliced
3 or 4 sprigs of fresh parsley, finely chopped
2 egg whites
1 egg yolk
½ cup cider vinegar
1 teaspoon Lite salt, or to taste
¼ teaspoon white pepper
2 teaspoons dry mustard
  Dash Tabasco sauce
1 to 2 packets powdered artificial sweetener
2 cups plain lowfat yogurt

Chop up all those veggies somehow or other. If you're a man, you'll find it goes a lot faster in front of the television watching football. If you're a woman, Oprah or Geraldo should do the trick. Mix up everything you've chopped and put it in the refrigerator to chill while you make the dressing.

Over low heat or in a double boiler, mix the eggs, vinegar, and seasonings except the sweetener. Cook and stir until it is thick and smooth. Then cool it and stir in the sweetener and yogurt. Add as much as you like or think you need to the chilled cabbage mixture.

If you have dressing left over, it is good on green salad or sliced tomatoes. If you think you've earned potato salad, it's good on that, too.

Charlene's Cauliflower au Gratin

4 to 6 servings

This is a pretty simple dish, but it's real good.

1 head cauliflower
¾ cup grated sharp Cheddar cheese

Charlene says to cut apart the cauliflower and place it on a steamer insert in a pot with about ½ inch of water in the bottom. Steam for about 10 minutes, depending on how crunchy you like your cauliflower. Then put it in a serving bowl and sprinkle with grated cheese. It's kind of hard to mess up this one.

Corn on the Cob

You don't really need a lot of butter on corn on the cob, although you probably have gotten used to it. Use whipped lowfat margarine and lightly trace a small pat over the hot ear of corn. Add a little Lite salt if you want to, but sweet corn is so good you may find you won't need anything extra.

Go into the garden and pick the corn. If you don't have a garden, find somebody who does. Barring that, go to a farmer's market where you know the produce is fresh and pick out the freshest looking ears, yellow or white. It doesn't matter.

Cook the ears as soon after you get home as possible. More than any other vegetable, corn begins to lose its freshness quickly after it is picked.

Shuck the corn, and pick out as many of the silks as possible. Heat a large pot of water to boiling, then drop in the corn and cover the pot. If the corn is young and tender, it should be cooked about 5 minutes. Drain and serve.

Do not leave the extra ears sitting in the water. If you want to keep them warm, leave about a half inch of hot water in the pot and put in a steamer insert to lay the corn on. It won't get soggy that way.

Corn can be eaten on non-Cheatin' Days if you don't overdo the margarine.

Ferina's Fried Corn

10 to 12 servings

Ferina is a feminist's worst nightmare. She still gets up early in the morning to cook Big Jack and Little Jack's breakfasts and iron their underwear. Then she hovers over them while they are eating to make sure they have everything they need. As soon as a coffee cup or tea glass gets half-empty, she fills it up again. Ferina also peels ripe tomatoes before she slices them and cuts corn off the cob. If you want to try this once, be careful. Your husband or boyfriend might get used to it.

10 to 12 well-filled-out ears of corn, freshly picked
1 slice bacon
⅓ cup water
    Black pepper
    Pickled bell pepper, diced

Shuck the ears of corn and pick them clean of silks. With a sharp knife, cut the corn off the cob into a pan. Fry one slice of bacon in a skillet until crisp, then remove. Add the water and corn, then cover. Cook on medium heat for 20 to 30 minutes, or until the corn is done, stirring frequently. You may need to add a dab of water. Sprinkle with black pepper to taste or serve with pieces of diced pickled bell pepper.

If this is a Cheatin' Day, go ahead and crumble the strip of bacon into the corn. If not, feed it to the Labrador retriever.

Fried Eggplant à la Fred

8 servings

When Louise left Fred to travel full-time with the circus, I didn't think the man was going to make it. He knew absolutely nothing about cooking.

I was over at his house one morning, and he was getting ready to boil some eggs for breakfast. "I like to boil my eggs about ten minutes," he said. "How long do you like yours?"

I said it didn't really matter, but I kind of like the yolks a little gooey. "Why don't you cook mine about three minutes," I said.

Well, Fred put his eggs in one saucepan, then pulled out another one for mine. "It was awful the other Sunday," he said. "I had three friends over, and they all wanted their eggs cooked different. I had a pot on every eye of this stove."

Fred's learned a good bit since then, such as how to put all his eggs in one pot, so to speak, and fish them out when the time is up for each one. He even went out and bought himself one of those Fry Daddys and a case of cholesterol-free cooking oil. Fred fries nearly everything now, but eggplant is one of his favorites.

 2 good-sized eggplants
 1 egg, beaten
 4 tablespoons cold water
   Lite salt to taste
 1 tablespoon black pepper, freshly ground
 ½ cup all-purpose flour
 1½ cups bread crumbs, finely crushed
   Enough oil to fill a deep-fat fryer to the proper level

Peel the eggplants and cut longways into sticks about ½ inch wide. Then cut the strips in half crossways so you have about a 3-inch by ½-inch stick about ½-inch thick. You can also cut the eggplant into ¼-inch thick slices crossways if you want to, but you get more seeds that way. You might try mixing them up, longways and crossways, to see which ones taste better.

Mix the egg, water, salt, and pepper in a bowl and beat well.

First dip the eggplant sticks in the flour to coat them, then into the egg mixture. Roll the well-coated stick in the bread crumb mixture (which you should have put in a flat dish by now), and drop into the deep fat fryer (which should be bubbling at about 375 degrees). Don't crowd the sticks, now. They will take only about 3 minutes to turn golden brown. Drain on paper towels and serve hot.

You can use this recipe for yellow squash or zucchini, too.

Uptown Upscale Collards

4 to 6 servings

Find a store that will sell you collards loose, not in those big bunches where the smallest leaf is as big as a Volkswagen. Yeah, I know it looks like you're getting more for your money, but all you are really getting is a tough vegetable that will stink when you cook it and haunt you long after you've eaten it. Big rubber-band bunches of collards are why they have a bad name.

Once you have found your store, find the produce manager, look him in the eye, shake his hand, and say, "You can't imagine how long I've been looking for a store that sells collards loose. Please don't stop." This may sound silly to you now, but once you've tasted these collards, you will want a continued supply.

> **2 to 3 pounds collard greens, loose, young leaves only**
> **Black pepper, freshly ground**
> **1 teaspoon Lite salt**
> **1 large onion, chopped**
> **2 cups water**
> **3 slices bacon, leanish**
> **1 to 2 tablespoons Balsamic vinegar (see note)**

Pick out only the youngest, smallest bunches. These are the hearts of the collard plants. Take them home, fill up the sink with cold water, and rinse them real good. Drain on paper towels, remove the leaves from the stems, and chop coarsely. If you like the stems, dice up some of the tender ones and add them.

Put the collards in a big pot with a tight-fitting lid. (If you've ever cooked collards or been around anybody who has, you don't need to ask why the lid has to fit tight.) Sprinkle with fresh ground pepper and Lite salt, and add the onion and water. Put the lid on and simmer.

Fry the bacon until crisp in a separate pan; drain and save the grease. Crumble the bacon and add to the pot, along with 2 tablespoons of bacon fat. Taste it as you add the bacon fat; you'll be surprised at how little you need.

Continue simmering until the collards are tender. This ought to take about 1 hour, not 2 days like some folks used to cook them. I don't care *how* your mama did it. Once she tastes some of these collards, she'll revise her recipe.

Adjust the seasonings to taste and add Balsamic vinegar to the pot or to individual helpings to taste. Pay attention now. To adjust the seasonings does not mean that you throw in a quarter-pound of fatback. Trust me.

Note: Balsamic vinegar is one of those wonderful things I discovered late in life, along with older women, artichokes, and trout fishing. You may have to go to a gourmet food store to find it. It costs almost as much as fine Tennessee Sippin' Whiskey, but it's near-bout as good. It's great as a salad dressing, as a marinade for onions, cucumbers, and tomatoes in the summer, or for almost anything else you can think of. *Not that,* Joyce Ann.

Marlene's Mustard Greens

4 servings

Marlene says you can use turnip greens or collard greens, too, but she's partial to mustard. So am I.

    2 pounds greens, washed and picked
    ½ cup water
    1 teaspoon Lite salt

1 teaspoon black pepper, freshly ground
1 tablespoon cholesterol-free margarine
1 tablespoon Balsamic vinegar
½ teaspoon nutmeg

Tear the leaves into smaller pieces about 1 to 2 inches square and place in a large pot with water, salt, and pepper. Cover and simmer for 20 minutes, or until tender. Drain and add the margarine, vinegar, and nutmeg.

Bubba's Batter-Fried Okra

6 servings

This may look fattening, but it's only about 150 calories per serving. When you combine a serving of this with some other vegetables, such as stewed corn and sliced fresh tomatoes, you have a low-calorie Southern meal that can't be beat.

1 pound okra (get the smaller, tender sizes)
Enough cholesterol-free oil for a deep-fat fryer
   (the personal size fryers are good for this)
1 cup all-purpose flour
1 cup milk
1 egg, beaten
1 teaspoon Lite salt
1 teaspoon pepper

Parboil the okra first, then drain and pat dry with a paper towel. Heat the oil in a deep fat fryer until it is about 375 degrees. (Use a cooking thermometer; but if you don't have one, just drop a bit of the batter in the oil. If it sinks, let the oil heat a little longer.)
  Make a batter by adding flour to the milk while stirring,

then add the egg, salt, and pepper. Dip the okra pods (now these should be nice and small, about three inches long at the most) into the batter and drop into the oil. Cook until golden brown, remove with a slotted spoon, and drain on paper towels. Like onion rings and French fries, okra is best eaten hot.

Another Fried Okra Recipe

6 servings

If you didn't like any of the other okra recipes, maybe you'll like this one.

- 1 pound small-to-medium okra pods
- 1 egg
- 1 tablespoon water
- ¼ cup all-purpose flour
- 1 cup yellow cornmeal
- 4 tablespoons cholesterol-free margarine or oil
- 1 teaspoon salt
- 1 teaspoon pepper

Wash, trim, and cut okra into ¼-inch rounds, then dry the pieces on paper towel. Beat the egg in a bowl with the water. Dip the okra in the flour, then in the egg, then in the meal to cover well. Drop into a skillet with the margarine or oil (oil won't burn as easily) and sauté for a couple of minutes on each side until brown. Drain on paper towels and season with salt and pepper to taste.

Oralee's Okra Fritters

Oralee says you can cook her fritters on a non-Cheatin' Day if you don't have any meat with the meal. Besides, they are good enough for an entree by themselves.

Cooking oil
1 cup okra, sliced into ⅜-inch pieces
½ cup chopped home-grown tomatoes
¼ cup cornmeal
¼ cup all-purpose flour
1 egg
½ cup chopped onion
Dash Lite salt
½ teaspoon black pepper, freshly ground

Pour enough cooking oil to fill the skillet 1 inch deep, and heat the oil until hot. Combine all of the ingredients, stir well, and drop by spoonfuls into the hot oil. Cook each fritter until golden brown, turning once.

This recipe will serve six people, unless one of them is Wade "Hog" Martin.

Bubba's Real Easy Baked Vidalia Onions

1 serving

1 onion for each person served
1 slice bacon for each onion
  Lite salt

Wash and peel the onions. Wrap each one with a slice of uncooked bacon. Sprinkle with Lite salt and wrap in a piece of aluminum foil like you would a baked potato.

Bake in a 375 degree oven for about 50 minutes. You think you can handle that, Roy Bill? These are real good with corn on the cob and grilled steaks.

Bubba's Baked Vidalia Onions

4 servings

I hope everybody is familiar with Vidalia onions. They are the real sweet kind that grow only in a small part of South Georgia. Be sure to buy only onions with the little sticker guaranteeing that they are authentic Vidalia onions. I don't think they grow with the sticker on them. I think somebody puts the stickers on after they are harvested, like a Chiquita banana.

4 large Vidalia onions
1 tablespoon lowfat margarine
⅓ **cup bread crumbs**
⅓ **cup grated sharp Cheddar cheese**

Peel the onions and boil them for about 15 minutes, or until the middle part can be scooped out. Chop up this part and sauté quickly with the margarine, adding the bread crumbs at the last. (You may need to melt a little more margarine; I won't tell.)

Put the whole onions in a shallow glass baking dish, and cover the bottom with a little water. Now stuff the onions with the sautéed mixture, leaving a little room at the top to sprinkle some grated cheese. Bake in a 350 degree oven for 20 to 25 minutes, or until the cheese is melted.

SueLee's Spinach

2 to 3 servings

Yes, I know you never eat spinach, even after watching all those Popeye cartoons as a child. Certainly nobody I knew wanted his forearms to swell up like Popeye's, even if he did have a tattoo. You're grown up now, sport, and it's time for you to try some of SueLee's Spinach. This is guaranteed to make you go back for seconds.

If you have a little garden plot, you really should try growing your own spinach. It's easy. All you have to do is dig up a little square in the corner of the garden, mix in a lot of chicken manure (this is not the recipe, now—this is just how to grow the stuff) and compost, and sow the seeds. Sow them in early March or late February if you're in the South. Spinach can stand frost and ice, actually everything but tornadoes and Labrador retrievers. If you don't have a garden, pick out a couple of bunches of fresh spinach at a farmer's market or a real good grocery store.

3 tablespoons low-calorie, lowfat margarine
1 pound fresh spinach or 1 10-ounce package of
    frozen spinach
Lite salt
Black pepper, freshly ground
¼ teaspoon nutmeg

If you have fresh spinach, take out the stems and tough leaves and throw them away. You will need about 1 pound of usable fresh leaves, so you will need several bunches. If you can't find fresh spinach, frozen will do in a pinch.

Melt the margarine over medium heat in a skillet and add the picked, washed, and dried spinach leaves. Add salt, pepper, and nutmeg, and stir. When the spinach is completely wilted, remove from the heat and serve.

John Thomas's Hoppin' John

8 servings

John Thomas doesn't claim to have invented this dish, but he did grow up on the South Carolina coast near Charleston where he swears he was eating rice by the time he was three months old. John Thomas uses dried black-eyed peas or dried field-peas in his Hoppin' John, depending on his mood. You can do the same.

4 cups water
1 cup dried black-eyed peas
2 slices bacon
1 medium onion, chopped in ½-inch pieces
1 cup long-grain rice, uncooked
1 teaspoon Lite salt
  Black pepper, freshly ground

Put the water and peas in a 2-quart saucepan, cover, and bring to a boil, then turn down the heat until the peas are simmering. Cook, covered, until they are tender but not overdone, about 1 hour and 45 minutes. Check before then to see if they are tender yet. You may have to add some more water while they are cooking, so don't wander off to watch "The Guiding Light" and forget the peas are on the stove.

When the peas are done, drain off the water into another saucepan and save it.

Cut the bacon slices into 2-inch pieces and fry over medium heat along with the onion. Remove onion when it is clear. If you're real conscientious about your diet, throw out the bacon drippings and the bacon; if you're in one of your cheatin' moods, go ahead and throw it in the pot with the rice and the drained peas. Add 2½ cups of the liquid you saved, as well as the seasonings, cover, and bring to a boil. Reduce the heat and simmer for 15 minutes, covered. Don't look in there now! Remove from the heat and let stand for 10 minutes before you take off the lid to serve John Thomas's Hoppin' John.

Fried Green Tomatoes

4 servings

If you have never tasted fried green tomatoes, you probably are one of those people who've never eaten boiled peanuts, either. Boiled peanuts aren't on this diet, so I'll tell you how to cook fried green tomatoes instead.

> ½ **cup cholesterol-free oil**
>   **(you may need to add a little more)**
> 3 **or 4 firm green tomatoes**
> 8 **tablespoons all-purpose flour**
> 8 **tablespoons cornmeal**
>   **Lite salt**
>   **Black pepper, freshly ground, to taste**

Cover the bottom of a skillet with cooking oil and heat while you cut the tomatoes (unpeeled) into slices about ¼ inch in thickness.

Pour the flour, cornmeal, Lite salt, and pepper in a medium-size brown paper bag or plastic bag and add the tomato slices a few at a time. Coat well, then shake off the extra flour.

Add the slices to the hot oil, but do not overcrowd. They cook faster and crisper if there is room between each slice. Fry until golden brown on each side and drain on paper towels.

Fried green tomatoes are like French fries; they are best eaten right away, or they'll get soggy.

Fred's Fried Green Tomatoes for Cheatin' Days

6 servings

Most of the time Fred fries his green tomatoes, it's for the noonday meal during the week. We call it dinner in the South. We call the meal we eat at night supper: Jesus and His disciples had the Last Supper, not the Last Dinner, if you need any more proof.

These fried tomatoes are so good that Fred sometimes cooks them when he has company. It definitely has to be on a Cheatin' Day, however, since these are about 400 calories per serving, unless you plan on not eating the rest of the day.

¼ cup all-purpose flour
5 medium-size green tomatoes, unpeeled and
     sliced about ⅜ inches thick
3 tablespoons cholesterol-free margarine
¼ cup brown sugar
1 teaspoon Lite salt
⅔ cup cream
½ teaspoon nutmeg

Flour the tomato slices and fry in hot margarine or oil for 3 to 4 minutes per side, or until browned. Sprinkle with brown sugar and salt, and add the cream and nutmeg to heat for two minutes while spooning the sauce over the tomatoes. Serve hot and stand back to watch the feeding frenzy.

Tommy Lee's Stewed Tomatoes

6 servings

You can use canned tomatoes if you want to, but I don't believe they'll be as good as fresh, red ripe homegrown tomatoes.

- **6 red ripe tomatoes, peeled and cored**
- **2 tablespoons low-calorie margarine**
- **1 tablespoon fresh basil, finely chopped**
- **Lite salt**
- **1 teaspoon black pepper, freshly ground**

To peel and core the tomatoes, drop them in boiling water for a few seconds until the skins crack, then dip them out and plunge them into cold water. The skin slips right off, and you can cut out the core with a paring knife.

Cut the tomatoes into chunks, then put in a heavy saucepan with the margarine. Cook over medium heat until they begin to look like stewed tomatoes. Add the basil, salt, and pepper, then cook for another 10 to 15 minutes. This is one dish you probably can't overcook.

Potatoes

The first thing most people do when they go on a diet is to cut out potatoes and bread. That isn't necessarily the best thing to do. Eaten by themselves, potatoes aren't that fattening. The half-stick of butter and three scoops of sour cream is what adds calories faster than Jester Moore can strip down a Studebaker.

Actually, once you get used to potatoes without the butter, they taste pretty good. And if you still have an unnatural hankering for the butter taste, try some of those artificial butter flakes, Molly McButter, that you can shake on potatoes along with a dash of pepper.

Lay off the salt if you can, or use Lite salt. Every little bit helps, and your blood pressure will thank you.

Meanwhile, if you want to go beyond baked potatoes, here are some recipes that will satisfy your craving for starch without putting a strain on your double knits.

Polly's Potato Patties

15 to 20 patties

1 large potato, grated
1 medium onion, grated
1 tablespoon oil margarine
Lite salt
Pepper

Wash your hands real good and mix together the potato and onion gratings, then form into flat little patties. Lightly grease a non-stick skillet with the margarine. Fry the patties on one side and then the other until browned. Add a dash of salt and as much pepper as you can stand. These are real good with anything, especially Sonny's Salmon Cakes.

New Potatoes and Parsley

4 servings

These taste best when you go out in the garden before the dew dries and scratch around your potato plants until you get enough for a mess. If you don't have a few rows of potatoes in your garden, you should have. If you don't have a garden or a neighbor who does, go to your nearest farmer's market and get the freshest new potatoes you can find. The ones about the size of a golf ball work best.

8 or 10 new potatoes (red-skinned), freshly dug
1 tablespoon corn oil margarine
3 or 4 sprigs fresh parsley, chopped
  Lite salt
  Pepper

Brush and scrub the potatoes well, leaving the skin on. Place in a medium to large saucepan and cover with salted water. Cook about 25 minutes until they can be pierced easily with a fork, then drain.
   Leaving the potatoes in a hot saucepan, drop in the chopped parsley and the margarine and stir well until the potatoes are coated. Salt and pepper to taste. Cover and serve hot with steamed green beans or any kind of meat dish.

Pauline's Low-Calorie Potato Salad

5 potatoes, medium size
2 boiled eggs, whites only
¼ cup chopped sweet pickles
½ medium onion, finely chopped
Lite salt to taste
Pepper to taste
½ cup lowfat yogurt
¼ cup lowfat mayonnaise
1 tablespoon mustard
Chopped parsley

Peel and cook potatoes until done, about 45 minutes. Drain and let cool for an hour or so, then put in the refrigerator. After the potatoes have cooled, add the chopped egg whites, pickles, onions, salt, and pepper.

Just before you get ready to serve, make the dressing by combining the yogurt, mayonnaise, and mustard. Stir into the potatoes. Sprinkle with parsley before serving.

Roy Bill's Candied Sweet Potatoes

4 servings

Believe me, when Roy Bill gets in the mood to cook sweet potatoes, he cooks sweet potatoes. This recipe definitely is one you will want to save for a Cheatin' Day.

3 good sized sweet potatoes
4 tablespoons lowfat margarine
¾ cup packed brown sugar
¼ cup water
1 teaspoon vanilla extract

Boil the sweet potatoes until they are soft, about 15 minutes. Drain and let them cool. (If you have ever tried to peel a hot potato, you don't need to ask why you should let them cool.) Peel and cut into ⅜-inch slices and put in a baking dish that you have coated with margarine.

While you are heating the oven to 350 degrees, put the sugar, water, and the rest of the margarine in a saucepan and cook over medium heat, stirring regularly for 5 or 6 minutes. Then add the vanilla.

By now you should have some nice syrup, so pour this over the potatoes and bake for 30 to 35 minutes. Open the oven every once in a while to baste the potatoes with the syrup.

Roy Bill's Baked Sweet Potato

1 serving

Roy Bill is even a worse cook than Fred, but at least Eleanor taught him how to bake a sweet potato so he won't starve.

1 good-sized sweet potato for each person coming to dinner
Low-calorie oil
1 dab lowfat margarine for each person coming to dinner

Wash, scrub, and dry the potatoes, then rub the skins with some cooking oil. (Relax, you don't get to eat the skins; this is to keep them from cracking.) Bake in a 350 degree oven until you can pierce easily with a fork; check after about 45 minutes.

Roy Bill's Baked Sweet Potatoes are good served hot with a dab of low-fat margarine, or just by themselves.

On a Cheatin' Day you can eat them with some roast pork or some of Wanda Sue's Valdosta "Veal" Cutlets.

Renee's Red Beans and Rice

6 to 8 servings

Renee learned to cook this low-fat version of the famous New Orleans dish after she married an ex-football player from LSU named Milo. I believe Milo is a Cajun, because when he was over at the house recently and I inquired about his employment status, he said he had just returned from an appointment with a personnel director.

"How did it go?" I asked.

"Not good," Milo said. "I told him for a job and he axed me no."

Renee really doesn't mind that Milo is not working. She says she just wishes he wouldn't keep playing that tape of 20 minutes of crowd noise after Billy Cannon scored a touchdown for LSU in the 1959 Sugar Bowl.

> **2 cups dried red kidney beans**
> 1 large onion
> 1 garlic clove
> 1 teaspoon margarine
> 4 cups water
> 1 stalk celery, chopped
> 1 ham bone
> 1 cup chopped ham
> 1 cup rice

Soak the beans overnight in water, then drain. Brown the onion and garlic in margarine over medium heat. Add the beans, 4 cups of water, and remaining ingredients except the rice. Bring to a boil, then cover and reduce the heat. Simmer for 3 hours or until the beans are tender. Add more water if necessary. Beans should be soft, but not mushy, when done.

Cook the rice in 2 cups of water with 1 tablespoon of margine. If you want to thicken up the liquid some, take a half cup of beans, mash them, and stir into the liquid. Serve over the rice.

If you want to have this on your Cheatin' Day, slice a cup full of all-beef smoked sausage and drop in about an hour before the beans are cooked. Renee says this is one of two things that will get Milo away from an LSU football game. I guess the other thing is crawfish.

Fred's Red Rice

8 to 10 servings

Fred says he didn't start out to make red rice, it just turned out that way. Getting ready to go on vacation, he tossed a green pepper, onion, and celery into a pot of rice, along with some tomatoes. Later he discovered this is a popular dish along the Carolina and Georgia coasts.

- 2 tablespoons low-calorie margarine or oil
- 1 medium onion, chopped
- 1 cup chopped celery
- 1 small green pepper, chopped
- 4 cups long grain rice
- 4 cups tomatoes, canned with juice
- ½ teaspoon Lite salt
- 1 packet artificial sweetener
- ¼ teaspoon cayenne pepper
- ½ teaspoon black pepper, freshly ground

Heat the margarine over medium-high heat and add the onion, celery, and green pepper. Cook until the celery and pepper are tender but not browned. Add the rice and stir. Blend the tomatoes in a blender and add to the rice. Stir in salt, sweetener, cayenne, and black pepper. Bring to a boil and cook for 6 or 7 minutes, then pour into a casserole and cover. Bake in a preheated oven at 325 degrees for 1 hour or until the liquid is absorbed.

Squash

It's hard to mess up a squash. You can squash it, stew it, fry it, steam it, and even eat it raw. I'm talking about good old-fashioned yellow crookneck squash, of course, although my wife is partial to the new variety of straightneck yellow squash. Easier to peel, she says. Why peel 'em, I say.

Pick the squash when they're about 6 inches long and nice and tender. If they are hard with big yellow bumps all over them, they're probably too old. But you can peel these and mix them with young squash for stewing or for a casserole. Once you get tired of yellow summer squash, you can switch over to acorn squash and butternut squash.

LyNell's Squash Pudding for One

1 serving

I think LyNell used to make this for Austell and the kids, but since she quit the beauty shop job and moved to Atlanta she doesn't cook as much.

    1 egg yolk
    ½ cup skim milk
      Lite salt to taste
      Pepper to taste
      Dash artificial sweetener
      Dash nutmeg
    1 small acorn squash

Beat the egg yolk with milk, salt, pepper, sweetener, and nutmeg. Add the squash. Bake in a small casserole dish at 375 degrees for 30 minutes.

Would you believe this only has about 165 calories? LyNell used to eat that many on the way from the beauty shop to her car.

Rhonda's Roasted Turnips

4 to 6 servings

I don't usually like turnips, but it is difficult to go to Rhonda's without eating whatever she's set on the table. The night I stopped by (to see her husband, naturally; it wasn't my fault he was out looking at his trot-lines), she had just made a batch of roasted turnips. They were pretty good. I may go back as soon as I find out when Robert Lee is checking his trot-lines again.

⅓ cup cholesterol-free shortening
4 to 6 medium turnips, peeled
Lite salt to taste
Pepper to taste

Grease a casserole dish with the shortening (or margarine) or place the turnips in there. Bake uncovered in 375-degree oven for an hour, turning the turnips once every half hour. Then increase the temperature to 400 degrees and bake for another 15 minutes or until browned and tender.

You may need to brush them with a little oil or margarine as they are cooking. Season with Lite salt and pepper to taste. They're not bad.

Sara LouAnn's Sufferin' Succotash

6 to 8 servings

Sara LouAnn is not a woman who endures misery easily. She will tell anyone who's interested—and many who aren't—about the latest ache and pain, catastrophe or dilemma in her life. Every time I stop by to see her husband Jack, Sara LouAnn is bending over the ironing board holding her lower back. She says cooking her succotash perks her up when she's feeling particularly low. Jack says they have succotash four to five times a week.

- 2 cups butterbeans (lima beans) or butterpeas
- 2 cups whole kernel corn
- 1 cup skim lowfat milk
- 2 tablespoons cholesterol-free margarine
- 1 package artificial sweetener
- 1 teaspoon Lite salt
- 1 teaspoon black pepper, freshly ground

Parboil beans for 10 to 15 minutes, then add to a saucepan with the corn and all other ingredients. Cook until the beans are tender.

Zelma's Zucchini Pie

6 to 8 servings

Zucchini is the vegetable world's answer to rabbits. Last spring I planted four zucchini plants, and by the end of the summer I had zucchini everywhere. We made zucchini casserole, zucchini pie, zucchini fritters, stewed zucchini, steamed zucchini, zucchini bread, and anything else we could think of. By August we were looking for ways to make jewelry out of it, but we had little success. What I'm trying to tell you here is, don't plant more than two zucchini plants unless you have a big family or a husband who is *real* partial to long, green vegetables.

Crust:
>   1 package dry yeast
>   ½ cup warm water
>   1 cup all-purpose flour
>   1 teaspoon Lite salt

Contents:
>   4½ cups zucchini, sliced thin
>   1 large onion, chopped
>   1 clove garlic, minced
>   1 tablespoon cholesterol-free oil or margarine
>   1 teaspoon Lite salt
>   1 tablespoon fancy white-wine mustard
>   1 teaspoon pepper
>   ½ teaspoon dried basil
>   ½ teaspoon oregano
>   4 egg whites
>   2½ cups grated Mozzarella cheese
>   Mustard

Mix the crust ingredients in a mixing bowl, knead, and let the dough rise for 10 minutes or so. On a warm day you can put it in the back window of your car under a dishtowel. Slice the zucchini into thin slices; you can peel it if you want to, but it tastes better with the peeling left on. Sauté the onions, minced garlic, and squash in the oil until tender, but not overcooked. About 10 minutes should do it. Add the seasonings. Beat the egg whites with the cheese and stir into the mixture.

Preheat the oven to 375 degrees and put the yeast dough into a quiche pan. If you don't tell your husband it's quiche, he won't know the difference. If you don't have a quiche pan, a 9 x 13 baking dish will do fine.

Spread the pastry over the bottom of the pan and up the edges to form a crust, then spread with mustard. Pour the squash mixture in and bake for 35 minutes or until done.

You can cover the crust with foil to keep it from getting too brown during the last 15 minutes of baking. Let it cool for a while before serving.

Desserts

Yes, you can have dessert on the Sonny Bubba Southern Fried, Semi-Low Calorie Diet, but you can't overdo it. No second helpings of chocolate cake or pecan pie with enough ice cream to open up a Dairy Queen franchise.

Brown Betty Lou

4 servings

2 cups sliced apples (3 medium) Granny Smiths or
  Golden Delicious
1 cup fresh bread crumbs
12 packets brown sugar substitute
1 teaspoon cinnamon
½ teaspoon nutmeg
2 tablespoons low-calorie margarine, melted
½ cup water

Mix the apples and bread crumbs, reserving 2 tablespoons of crumbs, with the sugar substitute and spices. Let it sit for a bit, then stir in the margarine and dump the whole thing in a baking dish. Pour the water over it, sprinkle the rest of the crumbs on top, and bake in a 350 degree oven for 45 minutes. Serve warm, by itself, ignoring the urge to cover it with whipped cream or ice cream.

Granny's Granny Smith Applesauce

4 to 6 servings

10 Granny Smith apples, peeled and cored
¾ cup apple cider
  Enough brown sugar substitute to equal ¼ cup packed
  brown sugar

1 teaspoon cinnamon
½ teaspoon nutmeg

Cut the apples into chunks and place in a large saucepan with the cider. Cook for about 35 or 40 minutes, stirring every few minutes. Stir in the sugar substitute and spices and cook until the apples have turned into a chunky sauce.

This is good with pork chops or Wanda June's Valdosta "Veal" Cutlets. (See recipe.)

Wanda's Waldorf Salad

8 servings

Yes, I know this is a salad, but it's a nice psychological trick to wait until after the meal to eat this, like it's dessert.

5 large apples, unpeeled, but chopped into chunks
1 cup chopped pecans
1 stalk celery, chopped
1 cup raisins
¼ cup reduced calorie mayonnaise
¼ cup plain lowfat yogurt or reduced calorie sour cream
1 teaspoon lemon juice

Mix all of the ingredients in a mixing bowl, pour into a nice glass serving bowl, and chill until ready to serve.

Earlene's Peach Cobbler

6 servings

Earlene says she wants it understood that this is definitely a Cheatin' Day dessert. You can use canned peaches if you want to, but fresh peaches are much better.

    1¼ cups sugar
    ¼ cup butter or low-calorie margarine
    1 cup all-purpose flour
    2 teaspoons baking powder
    ¼ teaspoon Lite salt
    ½ cup milk
    ¾ cup sugar
    4 cups sliced fresh peaches or 2 large cans canned
        peaches, drained

Cream the sugar and butter. Sift the flour and add the baking powder and salt. Add the flour to the sugar-butter mixture and pour in the milk. Mix well, then pour the batter into a lightly greased baking dish. Sprinkle ¾ cup sugar over the peaches and add to the cobbler. That's right, just pour the peaches on top of the batter. Bake in a 375 degree oven for about 45 minutes. As the batter cooks, it will rise up over the fruit and make a nice crust.

Rona's Raspberry Peaches

8 servings

You really do need fresh peaches for this one, but this is a dish you can eat on a non-Cheatin' Day, too.

4 cups water
1 cup plus 3 tablespoons sugar
1 tablespoon vanilla extract
1 tablespoon lemon juice
8 ripe peaches, unpeeled
3 cups fresh raspberries

Cook the water, 1 cup of sugar, vanilla and lemon juice over low heat in a large saucepan, stirring well. After the liquid starts simmering and all the sugar has dissolved, add the unpeeled peaches. Keep on low heat without simmering until the peaches are soft when tested with a knife. (This is about 7 or 8 minutes.) Remove the pan from the heat and cool for 20 minutes. Remove the peaches and drain. Peel while warm and put in serving dishes.

Mix the raspberries and 3 tablespoons of sugar in a blender until the berries are mashed good. Pour this mixture over the peaches and keep chilled until ready to serve.

Pauline's Peach Jello Delite

8 servings

Pauline says she started making this after all her friends began dying and she couldn't think of anything new to take to
the family's house before the funeral.

    1 6-ounce package peach Jello
    2 cups boiling water
    1 13-ounce can evaporated milk
    1 large carton Cool Whip
    ½ cup sliced fresh peaches

Make the Jello according to the package instructions. Add 3
ice cubes and stir until the cubes melt. Then you can add
the evaporated milk and chill until completely cooled. Add
the Cool Whip and peaches and you've got a dessert fit for
any funeral or family reunion.

SueLee's Strawberry Jello Delight

8 servings

Some people serve this as a salad, but you can eat it for a
light dessert. Besides, you need to have at least one Jello dish
to take to family reunions or dinner on the grounds at
church.

2 3-ounce packages strawberry Jello (you can use dietetic
    if you like)
1⅔ cups boiling water
  1 cup fresh strawberries, sliced
  1 small can crushed pineapple
  1 banana, mashed up real good

Dissolve the Jello in boiling water, and add everything else. Pour into a mold and refrigerate. If you really feel the urge, you can use low-calorie whipped topping when served.

Mary Anne's Mocha Mousse

8 servings

Before Mary Anne took one of those gourmet cooking classes at the night school, she thought mousse was something to put on her hair. As a matter of fact her husband Rory does put this on his hair, but only after an extended stay at Sambo's Road House.

  ¼ cup sugar
  ¼ cup unsweetened cocoa powder
  ¼ cup cornstarch
  1 teaspoon instant espresso coffee mix
  2 cups skim milk
  2 teaspoons vanilla flavoring
  ½ cup Cool Whip
  4 egg whites
  ¼ teaspoon Lite salt
    Thin slice of orange peel

Cook the cocoa, sugar, cornstarch and coffee mix in a 2 quart saucepan, gradually stirring in milk until smooth. Cook over medium heat until mixture boils gently, for about 5 minutes, and remove from heat. Pour into large bowl and cover with plastic wrap. Refrigerate until cold.

While you're waiting on that, beat up your egg whites and the salt in an electric mixer until stiff peaks form. Fold into the chilled cocoa mixture with a rubber spatula until all the white streaks disappear. Pour into 8 dessert glasses and refrigerate for an hour. Top with the Cool Whip and a sliver of orange peel, if you want it to look fancy and your mama-in-law is coming over.

This is only about 90 calories without the topping, so you can even eat this on a non-Cheatin' Day.

Lorena's Low-Cholesterol Banana Pudding

4 to 6 servings

This is almost as good as the real thing, Lorena says.

 2 cups skim milk
 2 tablespoons cornstarch
 ¼ cup brown sugar
 2 teaspoons vanilla extract
 2 bananas, sliced
 8 vanilla wafers

Heat 1½ cups milk in a saucepan over medium heat. Mix the cornstarch with ½ cup milk and add to heated milk. Stir in the sugar and vanilla and cook until thick, stirring often. Let the pudding cool and add the bananas. Pour over the vanilla wafers in a serving dish. Chill until ready to serve.

Lamar's Persimmon Pudding

6 servings

This all started back during hunting season when Lamar started bragging about what a great hunter he was. "Don't bother fixing anything for supper, honey," he told his wife, "I'll cook whatever I kill."

Needless to say, Lamar did not have a good day in the field. All he could bring home was a lardbucket full of ripe persimmons. Lamar says it's not bad, and a whole lot better than pine bark stew, which he had to eat on his last overnight fishing trip.

    ½ cup cholesterol-free margarine
    8 persimmons
    1 cup sugar
    2 eggs, beaten
    ¼ cup all-purpose flour
    1 teaspoon baking powder
    ½ teaspoon nutmeg
    ½ teaspoon allspice
    ¼ cup white cornmeal
    1½ cups skim milk
    1 cup grated raw sweet potato
    1 teaspoon vanilla extract

Let the margarine soften at room temperature while you preheat the oven to 350 degrees. Cut the seeds out of the persimmons and mash the pulp well. Cream the margarine and sugar and add the persimmon pulp and the two eggs. Beat this mixture well. Sift the flour and add the baking powder and spices, mixing well. Then add the cornmeal and mix well. Add the flour mixture a little at a time to the persimmon mixture along with the milk, also a little at a time. Now add the sweet potatoes and vanilla.

Bake in a lightly greased casserole dish for 1 hour, stirring 4 or 5 times. Serve warm.

Bubba's Bread Pudding

8 servings

        3 eggs
        3 cups lowfat milk
        4 tablespoons honey
        2 teaspoons brown sugar substitute
        2 tablespoons lemon juice
    1½ teaspoons cinnamon
      ½ teaspoon Lite salt
        1 tablespoon vanilla extract
        4 cups stale bread (just whatever you have left around
            the house)
        1 cup chunky applesauce
      ½ cup raisins

Beat the eggs and milk and add the honey, sugar, lemon juice and seasonings. Mix the bread crumbs, applesauce and raisins and put in a casserole dish. Pour the egg and milk mixture over this and stir. Bake in a 350 degree oven for 45 minutes. Serve hot with a spoonful of lowfat non-dairy topping and you've got a pretty tasty dessert for only about 150 calories.

Darlene's Depression Cake

6 servings

Darlene swears she's not old enough to remember the Depression. She says this is her Mama's recipe for a cake back when eggs and butter and sugar were scarce. It's pretty good and a lot lower in cholesterol, too.

     1 cup raisins
     2 cups water
     1 cup brown sugar
     2 tablespoons cholesterol-free margarine
     2 cups all-purpose flour
  1½ teaspoons baking soda
     1 teaspoon nutmeg
     1 teaspoon cinnamon
     ½ teaspoon vanilla extract

Cook the raisins in water, simmering until 1 cup of liquid remains. Set aside to cool while you cream the sugar and margarine. Add the raisins and liquid and beat. Add the flour, baking soda, spices and vanilla. Beat well, pour into a lightly greased square baking pan, and cook in a preheated 350 degree oven for 35 to 40 minutes.

Zelma's Zucchini Cake

12 servings

I thought Zelma learned her lesson last year when she planted 25 zucchini squash plants. She made stewed zucchini, zucchini fritters, stuffed zucchini, just about everything you can think of. Her neighbors started drawing their curtains when they saw her coming up the sidewalk with a basket of zucchini and pretended they weren't at home. Zelma made this cake for the Women's Missionary Union meeting one night, and nobody could tell it had zucchini in it.

1½ cups brown sugar
3 eggs (but only use one of the yolks; save the other two for an omelet or something)
½ cup cholesterol-free cooking oil
½ cup milk
1 teaspoon vanilla extract
2½ cups all-purpose flour
1 teaspoon baking soda
1 teaspoon cinnamon
1 teaspoon Lite salt
2¼ cups grated zucchini

Mix the sugar, eggs, oil, milk and vanilla flavoring in a large bowl. Mix the flour and other dry ingredients in another bowl and add to the milk and egg mixture a little at a time, along with the zucchini. Bake in a non-stick cake pan (a Bundt pan is good for this) that you have sprayed lightly with vegetable oil. Bake in a 350 degree preheated oven for 1 hour. Let cool for 15 minutes or so before removing from the pan.

Bubba's Bourbon Pecan Pie

6 to 8 servings

You can have this if it's your anniversary or you just won the Nobel Prize or your son just graduated from high school without wrecking the family car, getting arrested, or wearing earrings, or if your daughter married a fine, upstanding boy with no criminal record and a full-time job. Otherwise, don't even think about cooking this for an ordinary occasion.

5 tablespoons butter or cholesterol-free margarine
½ cup brown sugar (the dark kind)
3 eggs
1 cup corn syrup
¼ teaspoon Lite salt
1 tablespoon bourbon (yes, I know it'd probably taste better if you sloshed more bourbon on it, but just try it like this the first time)
1 cup chopped pecans
1 tablespoon all-purpose flour
1 9-inch pie crust, already in the pan (you can find these in the frozen food case at the grocery store. If your wife acts surprised when you tell her this, either she's a good liar or a good cook.)
12 pecan halves

Heat the oven to 350 degrees before you start. Cream the butter and sugar, beating frequently until the mixture is fluffy. Add the eggs gradually, beating after you drop each one in. Then add the corn syrup, salt, and (Um-ummm) bourbon. Coat the pecans in the flour and add to the mixture. Pour the filling into the crust and bake for 35 or 40 minutes, or until the filling is firm. Just before the pie is done, take the dozen pecan halves and put around the edges in a decoration, and bake for another 5 or 10 minutes.

If you want to serve this with homemade whipped cream, go ahead. Just remember that tomorrow is not a Cheatin' Day.

Index

INDEX   185